SURGICAL
TRANSCRIPTION
IN OBSTETRICS
AND GYNECOLOGY

Published in the USA by
The Parthenon Publishing Group Inc.
One Blue Hill Plaza
PO Box 1564, Pearl River,
New York 10965, USA

Published in the UK and Europe by
The Parthenon Publishing Group Limited
Casterton Hall, Carnforth,
Lancs. LA6 2LA, England

Library of Congress Cataloguing-in-Publication Data

Turrentine, John E.
    Surgical Transcription in obstetrics and gynecology/John E. Turrentine.
        p.   cm.
    Includes bibliographical references.
    ISBN 1–85070–512–7
    1. Generative organs, Female—surgery—handbooks. 2. Obstetrics—Surgery.
    3. Medical writing.   4. Medical transcription.   5. Medical records.
    6. Communication in surgery.   I. Title.
    [DNLM: 1. Genitalia. Female—surgery—handbooks.   2. Genital
    Diseases, Female—surgery—handbooks.   WP 39 T958 1993]
    RG104. T87   1993
    618. 1'059—dc20
    DNLM/DLC
    for Library of Congress   93-27723
                                                                                      CIP

British Library Cataloguing in Publication Data

Turrentine, John E.
    Surgical transcription in obstetrics and gynecology
    I. Title
    618

ISBN 1–85070–512–7

Typeset by H&H Graphics, Blackburn, Lancashire
Printed in the USA

Contents

Abbreviations   viii

Foreword   x

Introduction   1

Sample transcriptions   5

Anterior colporrhaphy   15

Appendectomy   17

Bartholin's gland excision   19

Burch retropubic suspension   21

Cesarean section   23
    Cesarean section for breech extraction   26
    Kerr Cesarean section   28

Cerclage   31
    Transabdominal cervical cerclage   31
    Cone cerclage   32
    Emergency procedures   33
        Saskatchewan procedure   33
        Wurm procedure   34
    Laser cone cerclage   34
    McDonald's cerclage   35
    Shirodkar cerclage   36

Conization of cervix   39
    Cold knife conization   39
    Laser conization of cervix   40

Dilatation and curettage   43

Enterocele repair   45
    Abdominal repair of enterocele (Moschcowitz operation)   45
    Abdominal sacral colpopexy   45
    Vaginal repair of enterocele   47

Exenteration   49
    Anterior pelvic exenteration   49
    Total pelvic exenteration   52

Fractional dilatation and curettage   57

Groin and inguinal node dissection 59

Hymenectomy 61

Hypogastric artery ligation 63

Hysterectomy 65
    Total abdominal hysterectomy 66
    Total abdominal hysterectomy with bilateral salpingo-
        oophorectomy 71
    Radical hysterectomy 73
    Total vaginal hysterectomy (with suspension of the
        vaginal vault) 76
    Total vaginal hysterectomy (with lash incision and
        morcellation) 78

Hysteroscopy 81
    Hysteroscopic ablation of the endometrium 81
    Hysteroscopic balloon tuboplasty 82
    Diagnostic hysteroscopy 83
    Hysteroscopic myomectomy 83
    Hysteroscopy for uterine septal resection 84

Inguinal and groin node dissection 87

Laparoscopy 89
    Adhesiolysis 92
    Adnexal torsion 93
    Appendectomy 94
    Bladder suspension or Burch procedure 95
    Cystectomy 95
    Diagnostic laparoscopy 96
    Ectopic pregnancy
        Ampullary suction and irrigation 97
        Chemotherapy of unruptured tubal pregnancy 97
        Salpingectomy 98
        Salpingotomy 99
    Endometriosis 100
    Hysterectomy 102
    Myomectomy 104
    Neosalpingotomy 105
    Oophorectomy 107
    Tubo-ovarian abscess 109
    Uterine suspension 111
    Uterosacral nerve ablation 111

Laser procedures 113
    Marsupialization of Bartholin's gland cyst 113

Contents

Vaporization of cervix   114

Vaporization of condyloma (rectal, vulvar, cervical and
    vaginal)   115

Vaporization of VAIN   115

Laparotomy, exploratory   117

LEEP (conization)   119

Marshall–Marchetti–Krantz procedure   121

Marsupialization of Bartholin's duct cyst   123

Microscopic fallopian tube reanastomosis   125

Myomectomy   127

Para-aortic node dissection   129

Paravaginal repair   131

Posterior colporrhaphy   133

Presacral neurectomy   135

Sacrospinous ligament fixation   137

Sacrospinous ligament fixation with anterior and posterior
    colporrhaphy and with complete repair of vaginal vault   139

Salpingectomy   143

Salpingotomy (linear)   145

Sterilization procedures   147
    Hysteroscopic silicone plug technique   148
    Irving sterilization   150
    Kroener method   151
    Laparoscopic sterilization techniques
      Bilateral partial salpingectomy   152
      Cauterization and transection of the fallopian
       tubes   153
      Spring-loaded clip or Hulka technique   155
      Falope ring (Yoon or Silastic band technique)   157
    Mini-lap Pomeroy sterilization   159
    Postpartum Pomeroy sterilization   160
    Uchida mini-lap sterilization   160

Suction dilatation and evacuation   163

Vulvectomy   165

Abbreviations

ACOG	American College of Obstetricians and Gynecologists
A&P REPAIR	Anterior and posterior repair
AROMED	Augmented rupture of membranes
BSO	Bilateral salpingo-oophorectomy (removal of both tubes and ovaries)
C/S	Cesarean section
D&E or D&C	Dilatation and evacuation (or) dilatation and curettage
EUA	Examination under anesthesia
EXP. LAP	Exploratory laparotomy
GSI	Genuine stress incontinence
LAVH	Laparoscopic assisted vaginal hysterectomy
LEEP	Loop electrocoagulation excision procedure
LFD	Low forcep delivery
LOA	Left occipitant anterior
LOP	Left occipitant posterior
LOT	Left occipitant transverse
LSO	Left salpingo-oophorectomy (removal of left tube and ovary)
LUNA	Laparoscopic uterosacral nerve ablation
MFD	Mid-forcep delivery
Monsel's	Ferrous subsulfate solution
MMK	Marshall–Marchetti–Krantz procedure
OA	Occipitant anterior
OP	Occipitant posterior
OT	Occipitant transverse
ROA	Right occipitant anterior
ROT	Right occipitant transverse
ROP	Right occipitant posterior

RSO	Right salpingo-oophorectomy (removal of right tube and ovary)
RX	Treatment
SCOPE	Laparoscopy (or) videolaparoscopy
SPROM	Spontaneous premature rupture of membranes
SPROM NIL	Spontaneous premature rupture of membranes (not in labor)
SROM	Spontaneous rupture of membranes
SVD	Spontaneous vaginal delivery
TAH	Total abdominal hysterectomy
TOA	Tubo-ovarian abscess
TVH	Total vaginal hysterectomy
VAIN	Vaginal intraepithelial neoplasia
VBAC	Vaginal birth after Cesarean section
VE	Vacuum extraction
VLL	Videolaserlaparoscopy

Foreword

The concept of a compilation of dictated operative reports and conversion of them into book form is intriguing and unique. To the best of my knowledge, it has not been done before, and is one of those things that makes you wonder 'Why didn't I think of doing that before now?'

Most of our medical expertise develops from clinical, on-the-job training with 'hands on' patient care, and no book, monograph, or journal article to guide your hand to ensure that you become a master craftsman, with the technique and skill required to perform proficient surgery. These come from experience in the operating room, under proper tutelage. This publication, however, may serve as a wonderful reference and guideline for the neophyte who needs a description of the game plan. It may also be of value to the more experienced surgeon – as a refresher, from time to time. How many of us have re-read our own old Op Notes on cases that we do not perform very often? If you have not, maybe you should.

I remember an old saying from my residency program: See one – do one – teach one. This is a catchy phrase, but, in this day and time, totally inadequate. I would offer: Scrub on a dozen, do a hundred, then teach. And teaching should be from a true desire and willingness to impart our art and knowledge to our fledgling members and professional colleagues, rather than, perhaps, some other less honorable motivations. Hopefully, this book will do just that, and be a helpful adjunct and catalyst in the quest for excellent patient care.

I have personally known Johnny Turrentine since his childhood, as a next-door neighbor, and then as a professional colleague at the same hospital for several years. He is a fine gentleman in all matters, and I wish him good fortune and contentment in the fulfillment of his life's dream.

Neal H. Newsom MD
Associate Clinical Instructor
Department of Gynecology & Obstetrics
Emory University School of Medicine

Introduction

I have spent the last several years developing, writing, and updating the following manual of *Surgical Transcription in Obstetrics and Gynecology*. When I was 'going through' the gauntlet of medical school externships, internship, and residency, I found myself learning how to actually perform surgery by reading about the procedure prior to the surgery, and transcribing the surgery. At the time I transcribed the surgery, I would often use an experienced physician's transcription of a similar case as a guide. I would change my dictation as to how the procedure was actually done. I would again read the textbook to make certain I had included all the information necessary for proper documentation. This method was quite tedious. I always wondered why no one would just research and write a manual of common surgical procedures to use as a guide. Many of my peers also felt a manual would be helpful.

I received my medical degree from the Medical College of Georgia, finished an obstetrics and gynecology internship at the University of Southern California/Los Angeles County Women's Hospital, and completed my residency at Georgia Baptist Medical Center in Atlanta, Georgia. I then spent several years in practice with my father who had 44 years of obstetrics and gynecology experience. I performed numerous videolaparoscopic procedures with Cameron Nezhat, MD, during the 'birth' of this technique. I then decided to move my family from the 'big city' to a 'small town'. My rural practice in the 'trenches' has provided me with the pleasant surprise of up-to-date technology and an extensive clinical experience. I have performed 35–40 gynecological cases and 20–30 obstetric cases per month for the past several years. I have delivered triplets, numerous twins including two sets just moments apart. I have faced many high-risk situations without the cushion of subspecialists. I have had to perform many procedures including emergencies without anesthesia coverage or surgical back-up. I feel my experience qualifies me to write this very 'clinical' manual.

I think it is important for interns, residents, and even clinical practitioners to be able to learn a type of 'form dictation' following their operations. Although every surgical operation is different, this book certainly does not include the complications and

1

unexpected findings so often encountered. The book has been researched carefully using standard academic textbooks, recent articles, and, combined with clinical experience, enables the obstetrics and gynecology physician to use this book as both a learning protocol and a guide to transcriptions for common obstetric and gynecological procedures. Many of the recommended transcriptions may be my preference and should not be considered the medicolegal standard of care. Many institutions may not be equipped with the technology described in this book. The book, however, is excellent for the beginning surgeon and can also be used by the experienced but tired obstetrics and gynecology specialist who might be dictating his operation in the middle of the night. These physicians would certainly not want inadvertently to omit some important aspect of their surgery that they automatically perform from years of training. This book should not necessarily dictate the exact form that should be transcribed but would certainly make an excellent guide to all obstetrics and gynecology physicians during their postsurgical transcriptions. This book would be important not only for more accurate medical record-keeping but important in reducing the medicolegal risks.

These surgical transcriptions should be *read before using the contents of this book.* There will be variation in surgical techniques from surgeon to surgeon. The importance of using this book solely as a guide should be highlighted to all obstetricians/gynecologists.

Many hospitals and institutions throughout the country have developed a number of suggestions and recommendations as regards to the methods of communication and 'how to' proceed with suitable dictations. There are very wide variations from institution to institution and each is generally a reflection of each hospital's recommendation. Many Medical Record Committees have come up with a number of suggestions which have been implemented at hospitals throughout the nation. When dictating an operative note, the typical format is:

(1) Date of dictation,
(2) Date of surgery,
(3) Name of patient,
(4) Hospital medical record number of patient,
(5) Pre-op diagnosis,
(6) Post-op diagnosis,
(7) Post-op operation (name of procedure),
(8) Surgeon,
(9) Assistant (s),
(10) Anesthesia,

(11)   Anesthesiologist (s) / anesthetist (s),

(12)   Drains.

The above should be included in all operative reports, followed by a section on:

(1)   Indications,

(2)   Findings,

(3)   Explanation of the procedure (technique).

The following explanations and sample transcription should be of help to any beginning intern or resident in obstetrics and gynecology who needs to be reassured that he is keeping up with the safety features, technology, and improved methods of performing and transcribing obstetrics and gynecology procedures.

There will be three sample transcriptions of some of my surgeries taken directly from actual cases. Form transcriptions will then follow and can be easily found in alphabetical order in the table of contents. I have also included an overview on some of the major categories and placed important points where I thought they would be helpful for the surgeon learning the procedure. I hope this will be as helpful to you as I wish it had been available to me.

John E. Turrentine, MD
Chairman
Department of Obstetrics and Gynecology
Hugh Chatham Memorial Hospital
Piedmont Women's Center

Sample transcriptions

The following are three full sample transcriptions. The remainder of transcriptions in this book include techniques only.

SAMPLE 1

Hugh Chatham Memorial Hospital
Elkin, North Carolina

OPERATIVE PROCEDURE

Name	**Number**	Sex	Age
************	******	F	25

Admit	Disc.	**Med. Record#**	Type	Room#
******	*****	******	O/P	0357

Date of Birth   8/17/1966   _____Physician_____
Physician   4201 TURRENTINE JOHN
Surgeon Dr TURRENTINE   **Assistant**
Date

Preoperative Diagnosis: Incomplete spontaneous abortion

Postoperative Diagnosis: Same

Procedure: Suction dilatation and evacuation

Anesthesia: General

Anesthetist: Foster, CRNA

Findings: The uterus was approximately 9 weeks' size. The cervix was already dilated with tissue and blood oozing from the cervical os.

Technique: Patient was prepped and draped in the usual manner for a vaginal procedure. Weighted speculum was placed into the vagina and a Sims retractor was used on the anterior portion of the vagina. A single tooth tenaculum was attached to the anterior lip of the cervix and the cervix was already noted to be dilated and enabled a #31 Pratt dilator to be admitted. Bleeding was very brisk and there was tissue protruding from the cervix. Using a #8 curved suction tip the intrauterine cavity was systematically emptied using the suction evacuation apparatus. After the intrauterine cavity was felt to be smooth and empty, a light sharp curette was utilized on the intrauterine cavity. Bleeding seemed to be decreased and the suction tip was again used on the intrauterine cavity. Hemostasis appeared to be excellent and a 4 x 4 sponge was held against the cervix for approximately 45 seconds after the intrauterine cavity had felt to be smooth and empty. The patient tolerated the procedure very well and all instrumentation was removed from the vagina.

John Turrentine, M.D./mt
D6-2392   T6-23-92

SAMPLE 2

Hugh Chatham Memorial Hospital
Elkin, North Carolina

OPERATIVE PROCEDURE

Name	**Number**	Sex	Age
************	******	F	25

Admit	Disc.	**Med. Record#**	Type	Room#
******	*****	******	I/P	0362

Date of Birth 6/08/1967 _____Physician_____
Physician   4201 TURRENTINE JOHN
Surgeon Dr TURRENTINE   **First Assistant** Dr Peterson
Pediatricians Dr Erlandson, Dr Groner, Dr Stuart
Date

Preoperative Diagnosis:	1. Borderline preterm labor
	2. PIH with Hellp syndrome
	3. Triplet, multiple gestation
	4. Primip breech baby C position

Postoperative Diagnosis: Same

Procedure: Primary Kerr Cesarean section

Anesthetist: Roger Gates

Anesthesia: Epidural (Jet)

Infant Statistics
Baby A: sex female, vertex presentation
weight 4 pounds 10.6 ounces, apgars 8 and 10, umbilical cord blood gas: ABG 7.25, VBG 7.29.

Baby B: sex female, presentation vertex, weight 3 pounds 12 ounces, apgars 7 and 9, umbilical cord blood gas ABG 7.20, VBG 7.17.

Baby C: sex female, presentation breech, weight 4 pounds 15 ounces, apgars 7 and 8, umbilical cord blood gas ABG 7.33, VBG 7.33.

Estimated Blood Loss: 600 cc

Technique: Patient was prepped and draped in the usual manner for a low Pfannenstiel abdominal incision. Incision was carried down through the subcutaneous tissue of the fascia. The fascia was incised with scalpel blade and extended in a smiling fashion by sharp dissection using the Mayo scissors. Overlying muscle tissue was sharply dissected away from the overlying fascia. The peritoneum was entered with sharp dissection using the Metzenbaum scissors and two hemostats to lift the entry site away from the underlying abdominal viscera. The bladder was then sharply dissected away from the lower uterine segment using smooth forceps and Metzenbaum scissors. The bladder flap retractor was then placed between the uterus and bladder to expose the lower uterine segment.

The incision was carried out using the scalpel and entry into the uterus was made being careful to expose the amniotic sac. The amniotic sac was entered and fluid was noted to be clear and there was no foul odor. Extension of the incision into the uterus was carried out in a low transverse smiling fashion being careful to avoid major vasculature along the lower uterine segment bilaterally. Baby A's head was lifted into view so as to expose the scalp in order to place the vacuum extractor. A pressure of 580 mg of mercury was applied in order to bring the head out of the uterus and with gentle pressure the remainder of the baby was removed from the uterus. The outer glove of the right hand which had been in the lower uterine segment was removed and the baby's oropharynx was suctioned thoroughly with the suction bulb. The umbilical cord was clamped in sections for cord blood gas analysis, routine blood testing and stat CBC to rule out twin-twin transfusion. Baby A cord was identified by one clamp at the end of the umbilical cord. The section closest to the infant was cut with scissors beyond the cord clamp and between the first clamp across the cord and then the infant was removed from the operative field by Dr Stuart. The infant was spontaneously crying. The second amniotic sac was easily visible and this was ruptured with an Allis clamp and found to be clear and without an odor. The head easily came into view and the vacuum extraction was placed on this baby's head and easily extracted. The remainder of the baby was delivered and the infant was spontaneously crying as the oropharynx was suctioned thoroughly with the suction bulb. An umbilical clamp was placed on the umbilical cord and then 2 clamps were placed immediately distal to the umbilical cord clamp for identification of umbilical cord B and then two sections of cord were clamped apart from this for cord pH, routine blood testing and stat CBC. The cord was cut between the umbilical cord clamp and the two clamps and the baby was removed from the operative field by Dr Groner. Debbie Myers R.N. was working with Dr. Groner and Luann Brooks R.N. was working with Dr Stuart with Baby A. The third amniotic sac was located and ruptured with Allis clamp. The fluid was noted to be slightly meconium stained. There was no foul odor. The infant was noted to be in a double footling breech presentation and an attempt at location of the fetal parts was performed for possible internal version but because of the small size of the baby and difficulty in location of placenta and multiple cords, it was decided that the best maneuver to deliver the baby would be by breech extraction. The two legs were grasped and in a corkscrew fashion the remainder of the infant was delivered until the shoulders were consecutively delivered. Using the Mauriceau maneuver the infant's head was delivered and it was crying spontaneously even prior to suctioning. Suctioning was performed, however, and then the cords were clamped with umbilical cord clamp and 3 clamps just distal to the umbilical cord clamp and then the cord was clamped into sections for routine blood testing, cord pH, and stat CBC. The infant was removed from the operative field by Dr Erlandson being assisted by Sandra Luffman, R.N. Multiple umbilical cords were easily identified by the one, two and three clamps and the placentas were then removed and it was found that baby A and B shared a placenta and baby C was contained in a separate placental unit.

Following removal of the two large placentas the patient was given several ampules of pitocin and the uterus was also injected with PGF 2 alpha to reduce the uterine size and decrease the chance of uterine atony. The patient was also given 3 grams of Unasyn IV. The intrauterine cavity was checked very carefully for any remaining products of conception and having made certain that there was none, the uterine incision was reapproximated in 2 layers. The first layer was closed in an interlocking continuous 0 chromic suture. The second layer was approximated over the first layer using a continuous limbered style 0 chromic suture. Hemostasis was excellent and the bladder was then reapproximated with 2-0 chromic continuous suture. After the uterus and adnexa were in the proper anatomical position in the pelvis, the uterus was inspected again and found to be very firm and there was no need for any further treatment for possible uterine atony. The abdomen was inspected and found to be in normal appearance including the appendix. The peritoneum was closed in a continuous fashion, 0 delayed absorbable suture incorporating the rectus muscle simultaneously. The fascia was reapproximated with 2-0 Vicryl in a continuous fashion. The subcutaneous tissue was closed with 3-0 plain on a large needle. Skin was reapproximated with 5-0 Vicryl in a subcuticular fashion. The incision was wiped clean with wet lap dry lap and benzoin was applied. Steri-strips were applied over the incision and then bandage was applied. Sponge, lap, instrument, and needle counts were all correct. The patient was given Duramorph epidurally and moved to the Recovery Room in good condition. The triplets were also in stable condition.

John E. Turrentine, M.D./pbg
D: 12-5-92
T: 12-7-92
cc: Dr Peterson
Dr Stuart
Dr Erlandson

SAMPLE 3

Hugh Chatham Memorial Hospital
Elkin, North Carolina

OPERATIVE PROCEDURE

Name	**Number**	Sex	Age
*************	******	F	24

Admit	Disc.	**Med. Record#**	Type	Room#
******	*****	******	O/P	0357

Date of Birth   8/18/1968   _____Physician_____
Physician   4201 TURRENTINE JOHN
Surgeon Dr TURRENTINE
Date

Preoperative Diagnosis: Uterine fibroids with pelvic pain and infertility

Postoperative Diagnosis: Same

Anesthesia: General

Anesthesiologist: Dr Justis

Procedure: Diagnostic fractional D & C with videolaparoscopic multiple myomectomies

Findings: There were two fibroids. One very large anterior fundal fibroid approximately 7 cm in diameter. This was on a thick stalk. There was a second smaller 12–14 mm subsersol fibroid along the right side of the uterus.

Technique: The patient was prepped and draped with betadine solution and draped in the lithotomy position with special attention to the area of the umbilicus and cervix. Weighted speculum was placed into the vagina so as to expose the cervix. A single-toothed tenaculum was placed on the anterior lip of the cervix and ECC was obtained in routine manner. Dilators (Pratt) were used until the cervix was dilated enough to allow entrance of a light, sharp curette. Intrauterine cavity was curetted in the routine fashion, until endometrial curettings were obtained on Telfa pad. These were passed off to be sent to Pathology. There was no fatty or unusual tissue noted. A single-toothed tenaculum was replaced with a uterine manipulator. The weighted speculum was removed from the vagina and the bladder was emptied with a red rubber catheter. Gloves were changed prior to the abdominal incision.

A small subumbilical incision was performed, and Surgiport Verres needle was placed in the incision and checked by the syringe, hanging drop, bubble and gas pressure register methods. All methods indicated proper placement of the needle. Pneumoperitoneum of approximately three liters of CO_2 was established and the Surgiport trocar was properly inserted in the abdomen. The sound of escaping gas confirmed proper location in the abdomen as the trocar was removed from the sleeve.

Videofiberoptics were connected to the laparoscope, and this was inserted through the 10 mm sleeve under videolaparoscopic visualization. Trendelenburg position was increased and approximately one to one and a half liters more CO_2 was allowed into the abdomen to better displace the viscera so as to easily visualize the pelvic organs. There was noted a large fundal fibroid along the anterior portion of the uterine corpus, and another subserosal fibroid along the right cornual area near the entrance of the fallopian tube. It was at this point that a second trocar was placed. A 12 mm trocar was placed approximately 5–6 cm below the umbilical incision, and through the 10 mm sleeve the stalk was grasped with flat duckbill bipolar forceps and carefully coagulated from all sides for approximately 30 seconds until hemostasis was thought to be assured. The myoma was then excised with laparoscopic hook scissors. Oozing was controlled with the flat duckbill bipolar coagulator.

The myoma was then placed into the posterior cul-de-sac with four-prong graspers and then thorough irrigation was performed over the uterine fundus.

The embedded myoma was estimated as to size and extent, and it was decided that there was no need for any vasopressin injection because it was felt that the fibroid could be removed using the flat duckbill bipolar forceps and/or point coagulator. The coagulation was performed along the outside of the serosa.

The fibroid had to be manipulated through the single puncture until the stalk was reached and coagulation was performed using the flat duckbill bipolar forceps. Once the myoma was noted to be white due to ischemia, the serosal capsule was then endocoagulated with flat duckbill bipolar forceps, and the capsule was easily dissected away using the flat duckbill bipolar forceps, establishing a clean plane. After the capsule was systematically stripped off the myoma using the coagulator, the myoma was stabilized with large four-prong grasping forceps and further dissection was performed with the flat duckbill bipolar forceps and then the base was reached and care was taken not to lacerate any feeding vessels. Nevertheless, there was still some bleeding which was unable to be controlled with simply the flat duckbill bipolar forceps. The pedicle was able to be cut with the hook scissors and removed, and then hemostasis was brought into effect by placing the laparoscopic flat duckbill bipolar forceps into the bed where the fibroid had been removed. The myoma was detached by twisting the pedicle with the four-prong grasper as the base of the fibroid was being coagulated with the flat duckbill bipolar forceps. The four-prong grasper was then used to place the smaller fibroid into the posterior cul-de-sac.

The crater was then thoroughly irrigated with normal saline and inspected for hemostasis. Interceed was placed over both the cornual crater and over the fundal crater. Extraction was then attempted by using the four-prong grasper and pulling it up through the 12 mm trocar, but neither fibroid would be removed using this method. A posterior colpotomy was performed after several attempts to split the fibroids. A speculum was placed into the vagina. Retractors were utilized and an incision was made in the posterior vaginal wall and the peritoneum. Immediately the pneumoperitoneum was lost, and also the fibroids were lost. Videolaparoscopy could not be used to see the fibroids, therefore, my hand was placed into the pelvis through the posterior colpotomy, and the fibroids were palpated. An Allis clamp was then placed between my fingers, and the larger fibroid was extracted, but the smaller fibroid could not be reached. At this point the colpotomy incision was reapproximated and hemostasis was brought into effect using interrupted interlocking sutures of 0 chromic suture. Hemostasis was excellent, and pneumo-peritoneum was again obtained.

Changing gloves the attention on the abdomen was again performed, and examining the abdomen thorough irrigation was performed throughout the posterior cul-de-sac with a Mandol/ normal saline sterile solution. The patient had also been given Unasyn 3 grams approximately 20–30 minutes prior to making the vaginal incision. The smaller fibroid was then grasped and the irrigation was thoroughly removed from the pelvis – the pelvis appeared to be uninjured in regard to bowel, vessel, bladder or ureter; the small fibroid was brought rapidly through the 12 mm sleeve as the sleeve was removed. With fibroid trapped between the fascia and subcutaneous layer, it was then grasped with a towel clip and removed from the lower incision. After assessing that hemostasis was excellent again, and that no injury had occurred to other structures, the pneumoperitoneum was again released, and instrumentation was removed under direct video visualization. Reapproximation of the incision was performed with interrupted suture of 2-0 delayed absorbable suture and placement of steri-strips and bandage was applied. Vaginal instrumentation was then removed, and hemostasis was considered excellent in the vaginal area too.

The patient went to the Recovery Room in good condition.

John E. Turrentine, M.D./lc
d11-17-92 t11-25-92

Anterior colporrhaphy (operation for cystourethrocele and Kelly urethral plication)

Technique

After the patient was in the dorsolithotomy position, the patient was prepped and draped in the routine fashion. A midline incision was performed through the vaginal mucosa extending from the apex of the vagina to the urethral meatus. The flaps of the vagina were dissected laterally with sharp knife dissection. The periurethral and perivesical fascia were mobilized widely by blunt finger dissection using a single layer of gauze sponge. Entry into the white appearing avascular plane just beneath the vaginal mucosa facilitated fascial mobilization, which was extended to the most lateral aspects of the urethral and bladder base. From a point less than 1 cm from the urethral meatus, successively vertical mattress sutures were made in the periurethral fascia. Bites were taken parallel to and on each side of the urethra to draw the fascia firmly beneath it. _____ (#0) sutures were used on a small curved needle. At the urethrovesical junction, the periurethral fascia was drawn carefully from its most lateral margin to add additional support to the posterior urethra.

The bladder neck suture began with a firm bite in the periurethral fascia. The suture was crossed under the urethra to anchor securely in the opposite pubourethral ligament high on the posterior aspect of the symphysis pubis. A similar suture was placed in opposite periurethral fascia and pubourethral ligament, which provided additional support to the posterior urethra and reinforced the high retropubic placement of the urethra. When the plication sutures were being placed along the course of the urethra and bladder neck, the assistant inverted the posterior floor of the urethra slightly with a Kelly clamp as each suture was tied. Cystocele was repaired by similar series of _____ (#0) plication sutures, which were placed in the mobilized perivesical fascia. The bladder base was displaced by a Kelly clamp and the sutures were tied in the midline.

The excess vaginal mucosa was excised and the margins of the vagina were approximated in the midline using _____ (#2-0 delayed absorbable) sutures. The adjacent fascia beneath the urethra and bladder was included in each bite of the vaginal suture so as to obliterate any dead space beneath the vaginal wall.

_____ inch iodoform packing was placed in the vagina. Instruments, needle, sponge, and lap counts were all correct. Estimated blood loss was _____ .

The patient tolerated the procedure well and hemostasis was judged to be excellent.

Important points

• Document evidence of uterovaginal prolapse or other indications (if present) if uterus is also removed at time of surgery.

• Document if injection of normal saline with or without vasopressors is used.

• Plicate the paraurethral and paravesical fascia *carefully* and *firmly* so as to elevate the proximal urethra and urethovesical junction to a high retropubic position. This action strengthens the circular fibers of the urethra.

• Many sources recommend using permanant sutures to keep the plicated fascia approximated long enough to allow secure healing.

• Leave enough fascia around and under bladder to provide a cushion of thickness to avoid entering bladder with suture.

• Dissect as laterally as possible to catch good tissue for support to the bladder neck and urethra.

Author's notes

This procedure is to correct *relaxation* of the anterior vaginal wall with or without urethrocele. Often multiple defects are present which must each be considered prior to surgery.

Removing a normal uterus to 'cure' incontinence is not necessary although many physicians believe that one achieves better success when hysterectomy is done in conjunction with colporrhaphy procedures.

Appendectomy

Technique

The appendix was delivered into the operative field by rotation of the cecum up and out. The vessels within the mesoappendix were doubly ligated with _____ suture then transected with particular attention directed toward the appendicular artery.

A hemostat was applied to crush the base of the appendix. The hemostat was then moved distal so that another small clamp could be placed just below the resulting groove. *(The stump of the appendix may or may not be tied with a ligature in this groove.)*

The scalpel was used to amputate the appendix along the groove. The stump was then inverted into the cecum using the hemostat that had been placed below the groove. This stump was then buried under a purse-string suture of 3-0 _____ (silk) suture that had been placed through the seromuscular layers of the cecum.

The entire operative field around the appendiceal stump site was then irrigated with _____ (kanamycin, neomycin, or cefamandole solution). *(The tagged sutures of the mesoappendix can then optionally be tied into purse string suture already closed.)*

(Describe the remainder of the closure.)

Author's notes

Often, the appendix is removed during ovarian cancer staging, C-Section, or hysterectomy. Many times, during surgery, prophylactic appendectomy may be done if fecaliths are found. Therefore, the benefits and arguments for and against McBurney incisions, paramedian incisions, drains, and other subjects associated with actual pathological findings will be omitted here. Technique of incidental appendectomy is described after already inside the peritoneum.

Bartholin's gland excision

Technique

After the patient arrived in the Operating Room she was prepped and draped in the usual manner for a vaginal procedure. After proper prepping and draping, the Bartholin's duct cyst was located and an elliptical incision in the vaginal mucosa was made as close as possible to the site of the gland orifice. This incision was made on the mucosal side. Utilizing Mayo scissors, sharp dissection of the cyst from its bed was performed. The cyst was mobilized further with the handle of the scalpel. The rectal wall was easily distinguished from the cyst by inserting a finger into the rectum during the dissection. This was performed utilizing a double-gloved hand. Following removal of the Bartholin's gland cyst, the vestibular bulb beneath the Bartholin's duct was located and the entire cavity was obliterated by approximating the walls with fine delayed absorbable suture material after excision of the cyst.

Hemostasis was judged to be excellent and the operative site was thoroughly irrigated with Betadine solution. Approximation of the vaginal mucosa was accomplished with a continuous mucosal suture of 1-0 _____ (delayed absorbable) material. The patient tolerated the procedure well and hemostasis was judged to be excellent. The patient went to the Recovery Room in stable condition.

Important points

- Broad-spectrum antibiotics are usually helpful during treatment of Bartholin's gland abscesses since these contain mixed bacterial organisms.

- Excision is usually a last resort after Word catheter placement or marsupialization has been tried, since complications include hemorrhage, painful scar formation, hematoma and cellulitis.

- Indications include persistent or recurrent abscesses or cysts. Malignancies need to be ruled out in postmenopausal women.

Burch retropubic suspension (Cooper's ligament modification of MMK)

Technique

After the intra-abdominal procedure was completed and peritoneum closed, the dissection into the space of Retzius was started using blunt dissection and only sharp dissection into areas of distortion and/or obliteration. Bleeding was controlled with pressure, careful fulguration and individual ligature, as was necessary.

The dissection was carried down toward the inferior aspect of the symphysis to within 1 cm of the external urethral meatus. With the patient in the semi-frog position and a #24 Foley catheter in the bladder, two fingers were placed into the vagina and the anterior vagina was elevated so that proper and accurate placement of sutures could be performed. Using the catheter as a urethral guide and the balloon as a spot for the trigonal and bladder neck area, sutures of #1 delayed absorbable material were taken into the paraurethral tissues and bladder neck and then placed into Cooper's ligament, avoiding any trauma to the periosteum. Two throws were placed on each side of the vaginal wall and urethra. Gloves and gown were then changed and the sutures were then tied and cut in pairs from below upward. At no time did it appear that any needle was placed into the urethra or bladder wall.

Important points (prior to closing)

- Suprapubic Silastic tube (#12 F) can be inserted through the skin and into the bladder under direct vision for abdominal drainage prior to closure of the incision. A small Penrose drain is placed on either side of the midline in the operative area if there is residual venous bleeding, and the wound is closed per routine.

- If there is any uncertainty about proper location of the suture along the bladder neck, the surgeon should not hesitate to open the dome of the bladder transversely in order to place

21

the suture under direct vision. Improper placement of the needle will probably cause symptoms of recurrent frequency and urgency.

- This procedure and the MMK are often the abdominal approaches to treatment of GSI as opposed to vaginal procedures such as the Pereyra and Stamey techniques.

- Remember that 80–85% of patients will have improved outcome no matter which technique is used and that surgical failures often result from poor preoperative evaluation of the etiology of GSI.

Cesarean section

An overview

There are three main methods of transcribing a C-Section which will be mentioned in this book. (1) The Kerr (uterine low transverse) incision which is the most common, (2) The Krönig (low vertical uterine) incision, and (3) The C-Section for breech extraction. Since the vertical incision still has indications but is rarely performed, and in light of the increasing efforts to encourage VBAC, it is only mentioned here. The C-Section for breech, however, still makes up 10% of the indications of why C-Sections are performed (according to National Center for Health Statistics National Hospital Discharge Surveys). Therefore, a sample transcription of both a Kerr C-Section and C-Section for breech extraction will be given.

Variations in technique to enter the uterus should be kept in mind. One may need to utilize Allis clamps to lift the small uterine incision away from the infant as the incision is carried deeper into the uterus. This can be extremely important with an occipit posterior position, where a facial laceration or orbital injury could occur. Scissors or manual extension of the incision can be performed and even using the Poly CS-57 uterine absorbable stable device might be preferred. (At present, information is limited on long-term follow up on patients and experience in VBAC when the stapling device was used.) If this type of device is to be used, however, it is just as important (or possibly more important) to insert a finger into the uterus to clear fetal tissue from the area to be stapled. The finger is then placed protectively between the stapler and the fetus to avoid entrapment of fetal tissue during introduction of the device. No matter what method is used to enter the uterus, it is most important to aim the extensions of the incision toward the fundus in order to avoid the major uterine vessels.

Infection and endometritis are the two most significant complications of the C-Section procedure. For the purpose of this book there are a few suggestions that might be recommended to include in transcription of the procedure. One should describe the appearance and odor of the amniotic fluid upon entry into the uterus. It is almost considered the standard of care to administer an antibiotic after cord clamping except in very low–risk patients. Some physicians prefer to give an antibiotic in regards to all C-Sections. There have been some sources of literature that propose lavage as an excellent prophylactic antibiotic (usually an example might be 2 g of Mandol mixed with 1–2 (normal saline). However, it appears that the less cumbersome intravenous method has become the standard of care for the prophylaxis of Cesarean section in labor. It is important to mention the type and amount of antibiotic used during surgery. There are many other methods that might help reduce the infection rate in each C-Section, including the removal of the outer doubled glove after it has been adjacent to the vagina during the delivery of the infant, removal of the scalp electrode before or during the procedure (if there is one present) and decrease of the number of vaginal exams *prior* to the procedure if possible. Some of these are certainly suggestions and have not been proven as an acceptable standard of care.

Removing the infant can be accomplished by the surgeon's hand, with the aid of a uterine head elevator, or with a suction device (Mityvac, CMI, etc.). If a suction device is used, the amount of pressure applied to the infant's scalp should be recorded. This amount should not exceed the following:

(1) 580 mmHg

(2) 21 inches Hg

(3) 10 lb/in²

(4) 0.7 kg/cm²

Infant statistics are often mentioned during the procedure or in the pre-procedure format. It is important to record the findings at the time of surgery so that this information can be easily retrieved if if needed at a later time. This is usually transcribed as follows:

Infant statistics:

(1) Sex,

(2) Apgars,

(3) Weight,

(4) Umbilical cord analysis: ABG _____ VBG _____ .

After the delivery of the infant and hemostasis is obtained, comment in regards to the appearance of the remainder of the viscera is important. A standard part of any C-Section is examination of adnexa, including ovaries, fallopian tubes, and related structures. Removal, to avoid probable torsion, is usually reserved for larger hydatoids. In general, because leiomyomas are vascular and likely to regress, one should not attempt to remove one at C-Section unless it has an easily accessible and/or avascular pedicle.

The abdomen should be checked while the patient's incision allows for adequate exposure. If the appendix contains a fecalith or appears abnormal, one should not hesitate to remove it. It can be embarrassing if the patient has acute appendicitis within a few hours after completion of surgery. The author has actually known this to have happened. One should transcribe all of these important points. The following pages give some sample transcriptions of Cesarean section dictations.

Important points

- Types of incision into uterus
  Kerr (low transverse):   most common
  Krönig (low vertical):   rare, but indicated in unusual circumstances (backdown transverse lies, etc.)
  Breech extraction: using either of above

- Variations of entry into uterus
  Use of Allis clamps if necessary to lift myometrium away from infant and increase exposure.
  Extension of uterine incision
      scissors
      manual
      poly C5 – 57 absorbable staple device
  Important points
      • avoid injury to fetus below incision!
      • aim incision upward to avoid major vessels bilaterally.

- Infection/endometriosis
      Describe appearance and odor of amniotic fluid.
      Antibiotic after clamping cord.
          Lavage or intravenously?
      Consider double gloving and removing outer glove that was in lower uterine segment.
      Decrease number of vaginal exams prior to surgery.

- Record method of delivery
      Hand
      Uterine head elevator
      Suction device (Mityvac, CMI, etc.)
          Record pressure applied

Pressure not to exceed:
(1) 580 mmHg
(2) 21 inches Hg
(3) 10 lb/in^2
(4) 0.7 kg/cm^2

• Record infant statistics
Sex, Apgars, weight, and umbilical cord analysis (ABG, VBG, etc.)

• Note:
Hemodynamics
Appearance of viscera
Exam of adnexa
Removal of any large hydatoids to avoid torsion but mention of any leiomyoma unless on an easily accessible or avascular pedicle
Appearance and/or removal of appendix
Closure

CESAREAN SECTION FOR BREECH EXTRACTION

Technique

Patient was prepped and draped in the usual manner for a low Pfannenstiel abdominal incision. The incision was carried down through the subcutaneous tissue to the fascia. The fascia was incised with the scalpel blade and extended in a smiling fashion by sharp dissection using the Mayo scissors. The underlying muscle tissue was sharply dissected away from overlying fascia. The peritoneum was entered with sharp dissection using the Metzenbaum scissors and two hemostats to lift the entry site away from underlying abdominal viscera. The bladder was then sharply dissected away from the lower uterine segment using smooth forceps and Metzenbaum scissors. The bladder flap retractor was then placed between the uterus and bladder to expose the lower uterine segment. Incision was carried out using the scalpel and consideration was made as to whether to perform a vertical uterine incision or a low uterine incision because of the abnormal presentation. It was felt that, since the infant was not estimated to be extremely large, a low cervical incision should be attempted with the idea that a possible T-incision be made if necessary.

An incision was made in the uterus in a low transverse fashion and care was taken to expose the amniotic sac. The amniotic sac

26

was then entered and the amniotic fluid encountered. This was clear. The extension of the low transverse incision was made with the surgeon's finger in a smiling fashion. The incision was opened to allow the surgeon's hand to be placed inside the uterine cavity. The surgeon's hand was placed into the intrauterine cavity and the fetal extremities were located. With mild fundal pressure the head was mildly pushed down and the feet extracted first. A towel was then wrapped around the legs and in a routine corkscrew fashion the sacrum was then delivered. Once the sacrum was delivered in a counterclockwise fashion, the body was delivered with very gentle pressure and then each shoulder was delivered in a systematic fashion, and then, in a smiling bite Mauriceau maneuver, the fingers were placed into the oropharynx of the aftercoming head and the baby was gently removed from the intrauterine cavity with both mild fundal pressure and the Mauriceau maneuver. The oropharynx was thoroughly suctioned with the suction bulb and DeLee suction. The cord was then clamped and cut as the baby's oropharynx was continually suctioned. The outer glove of the right hand, which had been in the lower uterine segment, was removed and the baby's oropharynx was suctioned thoroughly with the suction bulb. The umbilical cord was clamped in sections for cord blood gas analysis and routine blood testing. The section closest to the infant was cut with scissors beyond the cord clamp and the infant was removed from the operative field by Dr _____ . The infant was spontaneously crying.

Pitocin (2 ampules) was given in the remaining _____ of Ringer's lactate already infiltrating. The patient was also given _____ (antibiotic). The placenta and remaining amniotic membrane were then manually removed from the intrauterine cavity. The intrauterine cavity was checked very carefully for any remaining products of conception and having made certain there was none, the uterine incision was reapproximated in two layers. The first layer was closed in an interlocking continuous 0 (delayed absorbable suture). The second layer was reapproximated over the first and the bladder was then reapproximated with 2-0 (delayed absorbable) continuous suture. After the uterus and adnexa were in the proper anatomical position in the pelvis, the abdomen was inspected and found to be normal in appearance (including the appendix). The peritoneum was closed with _____ in a continuous fashion. The fascia was reapproximated with 2-0 (delayed absorbable suture) in a continuous fashion. The subcutaneous tissue was then closed with 3-0 (absorbable) on a T-26 needle. The skin was then reapproximated with _____ .

Bandage was applied. Sponge, lap, instrument, and needle counts were all correct. Estimated blood loss was _____ . The patient then was moved to the Recovery Room in good condition.

KERR CESAREAN SECTION (LOW TRANSVERSE UTERINE INCISION)

Technique

Patient was prepped and draped in the usual manner for a low Pfannenstiel abdominal incision. The incision was carried down through the subcutaneous tissue to the fascia. The fascia was incised with the scalpel blade and extended in a smiling fashion by sharp dissection using the Mayo scissors. The underlying muscle tissue was sharply dissected away from overlying fascia. The peritoneum was entered with sharp dissection using the Metzenbaum scissors and two hemostats to lift the entry site away from underlying abdominal viscera. The bladder was then sharply dissected away from the lower uterine segment using smooth forceps and Metzenbaum scissors. The bladder flap retractor was then placed between the uterus and bladder to expose the lower uterine segment.

Incision was carried out using the scalpel and entry into the uterus was made being careful to expose the amniotic sac. Amniotic sac was entered and the fluid was noted to be clear and there was no foul odor. Extension of the incision into the uterus was carried out in a low transverse smiling fashion being careful to avoid major vasculature along the lower uterine segment bilaterally.

The surgeon's hand was placed just inside the uterine cavity to gently lift the infant's head into view so as to expose the scalp in order to place the Mityvac suction cup. _____ mmHg was applied in order to bring the head out of the uterus. The outer glove of the right hand which had been in the lower uterine segment was removed and the baby's oropharynx was suctioned thoroughly with the suction bulb. The remainder of the infant was then delivered and the umbilical cord was clamped in sections for cord blood gas analysis and routine blood testing. The section closest to the infant was cut with scissors beyond the cord clamp and the infant was removed from the operative field by Dr _____ . The infant was spontaneously crying.

Pitocin (2 ampules) was given in the remaining _____ cc of Ringer's lactate already infiltrating. The patient was also given _____ (antibiotic). The placenta and remaining amniotic membrane

28

were then manually removed from the intrauterine cavity. The intrauterine cavity was checked very carefully for any remaining products of conception and, having made certain there was none, the uterine incision was reapproximated in two layers.

The first layer was closed in an interlocking continuous 0-delayed absorbable suture. The second layer was reapproximated over the first layer using a continuous Lembert style 0-delayed absorbable suture. Hemostasis was excellent and the bladder was then reapproximated with 2-0 delayed absorbable continuous suture. After the uterus and adnexa were in the proper anatomical position in the pelvis, the abdomen was inspected and found to be normal in appearance (including the appendix). The peritoneum was closed with _____ in a continuous fashion. The fascia was reapproximated with _____ (2-0 delayed absorbable) suture in a continuous fashion. The subcutaneous tissue was then closed with _____ 3-0 (absorbable) on a _____ needle. The skin was then reapproximated with _____ . Bandage was applied. Sponge, lap, instrument, and needle counts were all correct. Estimated blood loss was _____ . The patient then was moved to the recovery room in good condition.

Author's notes

This C-section sample suggested using a Mityvac extraction device. The surgeon's hand is probably the most common method of lifting the head out of the uterus. However, the vacuum extractor is *usually* the author's preference because of the seemingly smaller uterine incision that is necessary, thus decreasing blood loss.

Some sources have suggested placing moist laparotomy cloths in the pericolic gutters prior to making the uterine incision to absorb amniotic fluid, blood and meconium, in an attempt to decrease postoperative ileus.

Cerclage

Important points

- Contraindications to most cerclages include:
  (1) uterine bleeding
  (2) uterine contractions
  (3) chorioamnionitis
  (4) cervical dilatation > 4 cm
  (5) polychorioamnionitis
  (6) known fetal anomaly

Exceptions to the above can include emergency cerclage procedures during advanced preterm labor, bulging membranes, or when labor has been arrested prior to such cerclages (see Wurm or Saskatchewan procedures) – especially in rural settings when transfer of the patient to a tertiary nursery may be of utmost importance.

- Anesthesia is most often spinal or epidural.

- Make deep enough bites to reinforce but not so deep to rupture the membranes or injure the bladder.

- During the Shirodkar cerclage, many physicians have started tying their knots posteriorly to avoid erosion into the bladder.

- Abdominal cerclage should be performed only when vaginal cerclage has failed or is not feasible (secondary to the higher complication rate and need for two abdominal procedures).

TRANSABDOMINAL CERVICAL CERCLAGE

Technique

The peritoneal reflection was transversely divided and the bladder advanced away from the lower uterine segment using both blunt and sharp dissection.

The space between the ascending and descending branches of the uterine arteries lateral to the cervicouterine junction was identified. The area was developed carefully by blunt dissection medially to the uterine arteries and veins and laterally to the connective tissue of the uterine isthmus using long right-angle forceps with tapered jaws. The assistant provided upward traction on the uterine fundus so as to expose the internal os and tense the vessels.

After a 1–2 cm tunnel had been developed in the avascular space, the broad ligament's posterior leaf was punctured with right-angle forceps. A 15 cm segment of 0.5 cm Mersilene tape was passed through the aperture under direct vision so as to prevent slippage of the forceps or inclusion of tissue with ribbon and consequent laceration of thin-walled veins. The same was performed on the contralateral side.

The Mersilene band was passed around the uterine isthmus and over the posterior peritoneum at the level of the uterosacral ligament insertions. The band was flat, snug, and compressed the intervening tissue. The band was secured anteriorly with a single square knot and the cut ends were fixed to the band with _____ (2 or 3-0 fine silk or non-absorbable) sutures.

(Closure of peritoneum and abdomen is now transcribed.)

Author's notes

Pfannenstiel incision is recommended for 12–15 weeks' gestation but a vertical incision is advised thereafter. Transcribe the incision and entry into the peritoneum.

CONE CERCLAGE

Technique

Routine prep and drape was carried out with the patient under general anesthesia. A _____ (#16 Foley) catheter was inserted into the bladder. The cervix was visualized after weighted speculum and _____ (Sims) retractor was placed into the vagina. A single-tooth tenaculum was placed on the anterior lip of the cervix close to the bladder reflection and one on the posterior lip.

The entire ectocervix was injected with vasopressin (20 units in 60 ml normal saline) until the cervix blanched. Lateral hemostatic sutures were placed at the 10 o'clock and 2 o'clock positions on the cervix using _____ (2-0 polyglycolic acid) sutures.

A standard McDonald's cerclage (may transcribe complete procedure here) using _____ (#1 nylon or 5 ethibond) suture was then inserted as high and as close to the internal cervical os as technically possible without reflection of the bladder.

The cervical cone was cut using a _____ (# 11 surgical blade) with a marker suture placed at the 12 o'clock position on the specimen. Following excision of the cone, the McDonald's suture was tied with the knot placed anteriorly. A _____ (2 inch iodoform) packing was placed in the vagina and instrumentation removed from the vagina. The patient went to the recovery room and fetal viability was confirmed.

Author's notes

Cone cerclage in pregnancy was described in Am. *J. Obstet. Gynecol.*, **77**(2) February 1991. All patients are pregnant whose cytology or pathology is suggestive of invasive or microinvasive carcinoma, unsatisfactory colposcopy, or lesions in the endocervical canal for which the upper limits of the lesion can not be visualized and endocervical curettage cannot be done.

EMERGENCY PROCEDURE: SASKATCHEWAN PROCEDURE

Technique

After _____ (general or epidural) anesthesia, the patient was placed in steep Trendelenburg position. Routine prep and drape was performed along with vaginal irrigation with _____ (cefamandole) solution. Weighted speculum and necessary _____ (Sims) retractors were placed to expose the cervix.

Eight cervical stay sutures of _____ (#0 silk or Mersilene) were attached to the edges of the effaced cervix with a free needle. Care was taken to avoid the cervical edges with instruments and retractors so as to avoid perforation of the membranes.

Traction on the stay sutures was carried out to move the protruding membranes back into the uterine cavity.

Once the membranes are displaced upward, two rows of #1 _____ (silk or stout Mersilene) suture are placed as high as possible into the substance of the effaced cervix. These sutures are tightened and tied anteriorly. Half of the stay sutures are removed and the others are tied across the external os to close the cervix effectively. Vaginal instrumentation was removed and the patient taken to the recovery room in Trendelenburg position. She was given terbutaline sulfate 0.25 mg subcutaneously to ensure uterine relaxation. Fetal viability was confirmed in recovery room.

Author's notes

Traction on the stay sutures is carried out to move the protruding membranes back into the uterine cavity. If the membranes are not completely prolapsed, a deflated 30 ml Foley balloon catheter can be inserted into the external os of the cervix and the balloon filled with water to displace the forewaters above the level of the internal os. Once the cerclage is placed, deflate the balloon and remove the catheter. If all fails to reduce the bulging bag, insert an amniocentesis needle *suprapubically* or under ultrasonic guidance to withdraw several hundred cc of fluid to deflate the bulge.

EMERGENCY PROCEDURE: WURM PROCEDURE

Techniques

After deep general anesthesia was obtained and steep Trendelenburg position was achieved, the vulva was prepped with _____ (Betadine, Hibiclens) solution. The vagina was irrigated with _____ (Mandol or an antiseptic) solution. The membranes were gently pushed back into the uterine cavity with a sponge holding forceps (covered with a condom if available).

The assistant gently held the bulging membranes back as double mattress sutures of _____ (5 Ethibond) were placed from 2 o'clock to 10 o'clock positions and back in at 8 o'clock to 4 o'clock positions to be tied at 3 o'clock position. The next suture was placed at 1 o'clock to 5 o'clock and back in at 7 o'clock to 11 o'clock position and was tied at the 12 o'clock position.

Vaginal instrumentation was removed, the patient kept in Trendelenburg postion, and fetal viability was confirmed in the recovery room. The patient was also given _____ (prophylactic antibiotic).

LASER CONE CERCLAGE

Technique

After the epidural anesthesia was found to be adequate, routine prep with _____ solution and drape was completed. The laser bivalve speculum was connected to the smoke evacuation and blood evacuation system. The laser incision was outlined by short bursts of laser energy leaving a margin of 2–3 mm of normal cervical tissue. Power setting of 30 watts was utilized in continuous energy utilizing a spot size of 0.5 mm. The power setting was increased to 40 watts while lasering into the deeper areas of the cervical stroma. The cervix was blotted with an acetic acid solution during the entire procedure. The laser incisions were deepened to at least 3–5 mm straight into the cervical stroma, so that the cone could be easily grasped with several different pairs of laser Iris hooks to enable the beam to be angled toward the endocervical canal.

The conization was without complications and the cone easily shelled out so that the apex of the cone was able to be severed with a short burst of 40 watts of laser energy. (Some prefer to use a scalpel to sever the apex.) Following the removal of the cone, the 12 o'clock position was tagged with a safety pin. The cone was sent to pathology. The laser crater was then swabbed thoroughly with 4% acetic acid solution and bleeding points were lasered with 30 and 40 watts of power with a defocused beam and then swabbed again with 4% acetic acid solution. The entire crater was then soaked with Monsel's solution on a cotton swab and held against the crater for approximately 45 seconds. Hemostasis was _____ *(excellent, good, or describe blood control or loss – the following cerclage portion of the procedure usually also aids in control of any remaining oozing or blood loss).*

Utilizing a #5 Ethibond suture, this was inserted in the 11 o'clock position and brought out at the 10 o'clock position, brought around the 9 o'clock position and placed in around the 8 o'clock position and brought out about the 7 o' clock position, brought around the cervix and replaced at about the 5 o'clock position and brought out around the 3 o'clock position and replaced in the 2 o'clock position, bringing the suture back out at around the 1 o'clock position to tie with the original suture which was still in the 11 o'clock position. This was tied at the 12 o'clock position until the cervix demonstrated closure utilizing the finger.

Author's notes

Cone cerclage in pregnancy was described Am. J. Obstet. Gynecol., **77**(2) February 1991 and has been successfully adapted to 'laser' cone cerclage by the author, having what he believes to be much less blood loss. All patients are pregnant whose cytology or pathology is suggestive of invasive or microinvasive carcinoma, unsatisfactory colposcopy, or lesions in the endocervical canal for which the upper limits of the lesion cannot be visualized and endocervical curettage cannot be done.

McDONALD'S CERCLAGE

Technique

The patient was prepped and draped in the usual manner for a vaginal approach. A weighted speculum was placed into the vagina and utilizing a right angle retractor in the vagina, the cervix was located and grasped with an Allis clamp.

Utilizing a #5 Ethibond suture, this was inserted in the 11 o'clock position and brought out at the 10 o'clock position, brought around the 9 o'clock position and placed in around the 8 o'clock position and brought out about the 7 o'clock position, brought around the cervix and replaced at about the 5 o'clock position and brought out around the 3 o'clock position and replaced in the 2 o'clock position, bringing the suture back out at around the 1 o'clock position to tie with the original suture which was still in the 11 o'clock position. This was tied at the 12 o'clock position until the cervix demonstrated closure utilizing the finger.

This entire purse string suture was started anteriorly as high as possible and above the area where the smooth adherent mucosa covering the cervix joins the more mobile rugose vaginal mucosa. The suture was placed deeply, especially in the posterior portion since it is this area that most often subsequently pulls out. The patient was instructed prior to anesthesia that she must remain at bedrest for a minimum of a week following the cerclage and she was also given sedation and prophylactic antibiotics. All instruments were removed from the vagina and the patient went to the recovery room in good condition.

SHIRODKAR CERCLAGE

Technique

After routine prep and drape, a weighted speculum and _____ (Sims) retractor were placed into the vagina to expose the cervix.

The vaginal mucosa was incised transversely at the anterior and posterior cervical vaginal junction after injecting approximately _____ (20 ml) of 1: 1000 solution of epinephrine along the anterior vaginal fornix and posteriorly at the level of the uterosacral ligaments. The incisions are extended laterally about 1.5 cm on either side. The areolar tissue was separated bluntly by spreading _____ (Metzenbaum) scissors until the vesicouterine fascia was identified. The bladder was then advanced a short distance and then retracted. The posterior vaginal wall was similarly incised but care was taken not to enter the peritoneum.

Allis clamps were then used to compress the lateral paracervical tissue containing the blood supply. The anterior and posterior edges of the cut vaginal mucosa were then grasped and a 5 mm Mersilene tape swagged to double-armed tapered needles was passed between the blood vessels laterally and the fibromuscular substance of the cervix. The suture was tightened as firmly as possible while remaining flat and avoiding perforating the cervix or membranes.

Another high _____ (2-0 silk) suture was placed through the cervical fascia to secure the tape and prevent sliding of the cerclage downward. The anterior and posterior vaginal incisions were closed with interrupted 0- _____ (chromic or polyglycobic acid) sutures.

Conization of cervix

Important points

Indications of excisional conization (Pre-op)

(1) Lesion disappears into the canal

(2) Entire transformation zone cannot be visualized

(3) Abnormal cytologic smear in absence of positive colposcopic findings that cannot be explained

(4) Endocervical curettage indicative of disease in the canal

(5) Invasive cancer has not been ruled out by biopsy

LEEP conization is not included as this is most often an office procedure and not transcribed. (See LEEP for this type of procedure.)

- Specimens should be excised in a single piece whether performed with scalpel or laser.

- Twelve o'clock position is identified with suture or safety pin.

- If it is uncertain whether all pathology has been removed with the cone specimen, curette the upper margins of the uterine canal to rule out pathology above the upper margin of the cone.

COLD KNIFE CONIZATION

Technique

After the patient arrived in the operating room, preoperative vaginal examination was deferred and the routine intravaginal prep was not performed. The cervix was exposed with the patient in the lithotomy position and buttocks extended over the edge of the table. This was performed with a weighted speculum and a vaginal retractor. Lugol's stain was placed into the vagina and bilateral holding sutures were placed into the cervix laterally at 3 o'clock and 9 o'clock positions beyond the margins of the Schiller light epithelium. With traction on the cervix, the cervical stroma was infiltrated with approximately 50 ml of 1 : 200 000 solution of Neo-Synephrine in a circumferential manner. The cervix was seen to blanch and increase somewhat in size. An identifying suture was placed at the 12 o'clock position on the specimen with a single suture placed in the cervical stroma.

The uterine canal was then sounded gently and the sound was left in place to mark the course of the endocervical canal. A circular incision was then made outside the identifying suture and the Schiller light margin beginning posteriorly with the tip of the blade directed against the metal probe in the cervical canal. The specimen was then fully excised and the tissue was given to the scrub nurse and was sent in this condition to Pathology, being careful not to place the tissue in fixative at this time.

Sturmdorf sutures were then placed in the posterior lip first, utilizing a #1 _____ (delayed absorbable) suture on a large cutting needle. The suture was placed so as to pick up the posterior flap of the mucosa in the midline near the edge and then the suture was directed high into the endocervical canal passing through the wall of the cervical canal out through the portio of the posterior cervical lip near the fornia approximately 2 cm from the site of the initial suture. As the mucosal flap was pulled forward, the other end of the suture was threaded into the cutting needle and the process of suturing through the cervical canal was repeated. The two ends of the suture emerged on the posterior surface of the cervix approximately 0.5 cm apart. Firm traction on this suture pulled the posterior mucosal flap well into the newly made cervical canal and the suture was tied and the procedure was repeated on the anterior lip.

Superficial electrocoagulation of the bleeding points in the cervical stroma was performed followed by application of gelfoam sponge to necessary cervical defects. This was held in place with a vaginal pack which will be removed in approximately 24 hours. Hemostasis was judged to be excellent during the entire procedure.

LASER CONIZATION OF CERVIX

Technique

Patient was placed on the operating room table in the lithotomy position and, following careful pelvic exam, the laser speculum was placed into the vagina and the cervix was swabbed thoroughly with 4% acetic acid solution. The paracervical anesthetic was placed at 8 o'clock, 4 o'clock and 12 o'clock positions and the laser bivalve speculum was connected to the smoke evacuation and blood evacuating system. The laser incision was outlined by short bursts of laser energy leaving a margin of 2–3 mm of normal cervical tissue. Power setting of 30 watts was utilized in continuous energy utilizing a spot size of 0.5 mm. The power setting was increased to 40 watts while lasering into the deeper areas of the cervical stroma. The cervix was blotted with an acetic acid solution during the entire procedure. The laser incisions were deepened to at least 3–5 mm straight into the cervical stroma so that the cone could be easily grasped with several different pairs of laser Iris hooks so as to enable the beam to be angled toward the endocervical canal.

The conization was without complications and the cone easily shelled out so that the apex of the cone was able to be severed with a short burst of 40 watts of laser energy. (Some prefer to use a scalpel to sever the apex.) Following the removal of the cone, the 12 o'clock position was tagged with a safety pin. The cone was sent to pathology. The laser crater was then swabbed thoroughly with 4% acetic acid solution and bleeding points were lasered with 30 and 40 watts of power with a defocused beam and then swabbed again with 4% acetic acid solution. The entire crater was then soaked with Monsel's solution on a cotton swab and held against the crater for approximately 45 seconds. Hemostasis was excellent. Q-tips were also used to bring about excellent hemostasis.

The patient has been given routine outpatient laser instructions and will be seen in approximately 12 weeks for follow-up cytology and possible colposcopy.

Dilatation and curettage

Technique

Patient was placed on the operating table in the lithotomy position. Careful pelvic examination was performed to locate the position of the uterine corpus. The vagina and the perineum were cleaned with _____ in the routine fashion.

The cervix was grasped with tenaculum and gently drawn toward the vaginal outlet. A small curette was utilized to obtain endocervical curettings. These were obtained on Telfa pad and handed off to be sent to Pathology. A sound was then passed through the cervical canal into the uterine cavity. This was done carefully to avoid creating a false passage. The length of the uterine cavity was _____ cm. Once the position of the uterus, the length of the uterine cavity, angulation between the cervical canal and uterine cavity had been ascertained, the sound was removed and the cervical canal was dilated with a small dilator. After a 3 mm dilator was passed, successively larger ones were used. After dilatation of 9 mm was reached, the dilatation was discontinued.

A gauze was placed into the posterior vaginal fornix along with posterior weighted speculum retractor with a Telfa pad on top of the sponge so that blood and endometrium removed from the uterus would fall onto it. The uterine cavity was explored initially in search of any endometrial polyps with the polyp forceps. The forceps were moved systematically across the dome of the uterus and the anterior and posterior walls. The procedure was repeated several times and then the curettage was performed with a sharp curette. This was performed in a systematic manner in which the area of the endometrial cavity was covered. The procedure utilizing the polyp forceps was again repeated several times after the uterine wall had been curetted to make certain that there was no area of endometrial cavity that polyp or pathology might have been missed. A malleable, bluntly serrated curette was then introduced again into the uterus and in a systematic manner the entire uterine cavity was curetted. Anterior, lateral and posterior walls were scraped gently but firmly and finally the top of the cavity was scraped with a side-to-side movement. After appropriate endometrial curettings had been obtained, these were placed

43

immediately in fixative, being careful not to mash or scrape the specimens. There was no fatty tissue or unusual tissue noted. Hemostasis was judged to be excellent and all instrumentation was removed from the vagina and the patient was removed to the recovery room in good condition.

Important points

- ECC is usually performed with Kevorkian curette up to the internal os usually at least two times around with short, firm strokes, without catching portions of external os.

- Sound the uterus *only after ECC* to avoid pushing tissue from the cervix into the uterus.

- Try to predict severe retroversion so as to avoid easy perforation.

- Remember to note whether or not abnormal tissue was present.

Enterocele repair

ABDOMINAL REPAIR OF ENTEROCELE (MOSCHCOWITZ OPERATION)

Technique

With the patient in Trendelenburg position, the intestines were held back with damp packs for optimal exposure.

A purse-string suture using #0 _____ (silk or delayed absorbable) suture was placed around the base of the sac to encircle the cul-de-sac of Douglas. The peritoneum was picked up in each bite taking only light superficial bites into the serosa of the rectum. Successive purse-string sutures were placed until the uterosacral ligaments were reached then very firm bites were placed along these ligaments and the posterior surface of the vagina. The last suture was placed without undue tension.

The anatomical defect was completely obliterated without inclusion or injury to ureters.

Author's notes

If the uterus is retained, it is held up and forward with a traction suture. If the uterus is absent, the posterior wall of the vaginal vault is held under traction with Allis clamps.

ABDOMINAL SACRAL COLPOPEXY

Technique

The patient was prepped and draped in the usual manner in the lithotomy position with legs in place. Pelvic examination was performed and the vaginal vault demonstrated the defects of lack of vaginal support. (There appeared to be very little, if any rectocele component, and the bladder seemed to be well supported. Most of the prolapse was along the posterior aspect of the vagina with an enterocele component.)

After the patient was prepped with Betadine from the lower ribcage and the entire abdomen, anterior thighs, perineum, vagina, and perianal area, the patient was draped to allow easy access to the vagina and lower abdomen. Foley catheter was placed after the Betadine prep. A sponge stick with two 4 x 4 sponges was placed into the vagina and covered with sterile drapes.

A _____ abdominal incision was performed and carried down through the subcutaneous tissue to the fascia. Hemostasis was brought about using electrocautery. The fascia was incised and, using a sterile measuring device, a 2.5 x 10 cm strip of fascia was excised along the fascial incision and placed between sponges moistened with saline. The peritoneal cavity was entered using hemostats and Metzenbaum scissors. The upper abdomen was explored. The bowel and viscera were placed up into the upper abdomen and a Balfour self-retaining retractor was inserted. The sponge forceps were then manipulated through the introitus so that the vaginal cuff could be elevated and the vaginal apex could be observed very easily in the pelvis. Allis forceps were used to grasp each lateral angle of the vagina and the vesical peritoneum overlying the vaginal apex was incised. The bladder was freed from the anterior vaginal wall and the rectum was freed from the posterior vaginal wall so that at least 3–4 cm of vaginal wall could be noted in the apex exposed. The edges of the vaginal mucosa were approximated from side to side with #2-0 delayed absorbable sutures. Some of the peritoneum and its lining were excised along with excess posterior vaginal wall and further obliterated by the Moschcowitz culdoplasty using #2-0 Prolene suture. Care was taken to pick up the uterosacral ligaments with each bite. Care was also taken to avoid placing the suture too deep so that the ureter could be avoided. Four #2-0 figure-of-eight Tevdek sutures were placed in the thickness of the vaginal wall at the apex in a single row from one lateral fornix to the other. The graft was slid down the sutures to the vaginal apex and the sutures were then tied and cut. A second row of #2-0 Vicryl sutures was then placed through the graft and into the posterior vaginal wall near the apex.

The completion of the Moschcowitz culdoplasty was completed using #2-0 Tevdek beginning at the bottom of the cul-de-sac, and exercising care to include remnants of uterosacral ligaments in the posterior vagina but only peritoneum laterally. Only shallow bites of serosa of the sigmoid colon were carried out. There were no defects during the closure of the cul-de-sac that appeared could cause any bowel entrapment. There were no constrictions on the sigmoid colon.

With the sigmoid colon retracted to the left, the posterior and parietal peritoneum overlaying the anterior sacrum, was opened longitudinally in the middle from the sacral promontory caudally to a point below S-3. The posterior sacral fascia was exposed by blunt and sharp dissection exercising care to avoid injury to the pre-sacral vessels. There was a small amount of bleeding in one vessel which was electrocoagulated. Three permanent sutures of #2-0 Tevdek were placed in the periosteum of the sacrum about 1 cm apart in the midline overlying S1 and S4 vertebra. #2-0 Vicryl sutures were also utilized in between these sutures and these were on MO-4 needles and could obtain deeper bites into the periosteum of the sacrum. The fascial graft that was attached to the vaginal apex was measured and trimmed to reach the exposed anterior sacrum without tension. The sutures in the sacrum were then placed securely in the sacral end in the fascial graft and then tied. The graft segments were sutured to underlying sigmoid serosa and culdoplasty peritoneum to avoid any bridging between the graft and underlying tissues. This was performed with 2-0 chromic suture. The area was irrigated very thoroughly and the retroperitoneal space was reapproximated with 2-0 delayed absorbable suture.

The peritoneum was closed with #2-0 delayed absorbable suture. (The space of Retzius was not entered because an anterior repair had already previously been performed and the patient had not complained of any urinary symptoms.) A #2-0 Prolene suture was placed in a continuous suture in the fascia to approximate closing the incision. The subcutaneous tissue was closed with 3-0 plain suture after irrigation and after placing two interrupted sutures of 2-0 Vicryl in each side of the fascia following the Prolene closure. Skin was reapproximated with 5-0 Vicryl in a continuous subcuticular fashion and the incision was wiped clean with a wet lap/dry lap and benzoin applied. Steri-strips were applied and then bandage was applied.

Following placement of the bandage over the abdominal skin closure, the vaginal area was examined again. (It was noted that there would be no need for posterior colporrhaphy in that there was very little, if any, rectocele component.) The correction of vaginal prolapse and correct angle was noted to be excellent following the colpopexy. The 4 x 4 sponges were removed before and after inspection of the vagina. The patient was then removed to the recovery room in good condition. Estimated blood loss was approximately _____.

VAGINAL REPAIR OF ENTEROCELE

Technique

After prep and drape, a midline incision was performed posteriorly as in a posterior colporrhaphy. A tunnel was made beneath the vaginal mucosa using Metzenbaum scissors then the vagina was incised in the midline. The vagina was dissected laterally until rectocele component was exposed on both sides and the enterocele presented itself as a peritoneal pouch.

The enterocele sac was dissected free using blunt and sharp dissection. A purse-string suture using #10 _____ (silk or delayed-absorbable) suture was placed on the outside of the sac at the neck. The purse-string suture was placed along the inside of the sac above the levator hiatus. An additional purse-string suture above the initial suture was also placed incorporating bites into the uterosacral ligaments and providing additional support to the hernial repair. After all the purse-strings were tied, the margins of the sac were trimmed.

The posterior margin of the vagina was then pulled forward to place maximum tension on the uterosacral ligaments. The ligaments were approximated in the midline with two interrupted sutures that included a bite of the stump of the ligated hernial sac.

Author's notes

This procedure provides a firm new base for the cul-de-sac but if a rectocele, cystocele, or relaxed vaginal outlet is present, it should be repaired prior to completion of closure.

Exenteration

ANTERIOR PELVIC EXENTERATION

Exploratory laparotomy, radical hysterectomy, radical cystectomy, bilateral salpingo-oophorectomy, peri-aortic and pelvic lymph node dissection, peri-aortic lymph adenectomy, bilateral, pelvic lymph adenectomy, bilateral, ileoconduit formation, examination under anesthesia are included for completeness.

Technique

After intermittent venous calf compression booties had been attached, a satisfactory level of general endotracheal anesthesia was induced and examination under anesthesia was carried out. Foley catheter was inserted into the bladder and noted to return clear urine. The findings of examination under anesthesia are as dictated above. She was placed supine and prepped and draped in a sterile fashion. The abdomen was entered through a midline incision, extending up just to the left of the umbilicus. Exploration was carried out, all of the upper abdominal viscera were normal to palpation. There was no adenopathy appreciated. Exploration was carried out with the findings as noted above, i.e. tumor in the vesicovaginal septum. The aortic nodes were negative for metastatic disease; therefore, it was felt advisable to proceed with anterior pelvic exenteration which was accomplished as follows.

A self-retaining retractor had been placed and the bowels had been packed away superiorly. The pelvic spaces were opened by first dividing the round ligaments bilaterally with an LDS CO_2 power device. The peritoneum overlying the bladder was incised high to the anterior parietal peritoneum and then the peritoneum in this area was dissected down and freed off of the bladder surface so the peritoneum could be used for reconstruction of the pelvic floor later. The actual muscularis of the dome of the bladder was left to go with the surgical specimen to be extrapolated. The peri-vesical and peri-rectal spaces were developed bilaterally down to the level of the levator muscles of the pelvic floor. The rectovaginal system was opened and explored and found to be free of tumor. The posterior vagina looked as though it had not been encroached upon, therefore it was elected to proceed with anterior exenteration only. The rectovaginal septum was dissected down the length of the vagina and the colon pushed away posteriorly. An identical technique was used for management of the pelvic wall space and I will describe it in detail for the right side. Also described in detail below for the right side only is dissection of the ureter down to the area near the trigone. An identical operative technique was used on the contralateral side.

The right distal obliterated hypogastric artery was identified and the origin of the uterine artery from the more proximal internal iliac artery was identified. The soft tissues between the paravesical and pararectal spaces were mobilized. Dissection was then carried around anteriorly into the space of Retzius and the bladder was released from the infrapubic area. Blunt and sharp dissection was used to free up all the areolar tissue involved in the area of dissection. The course of the ureter was carefully identified and it was dissected down to the area where it coursed into the ureteric tunnel underneath the cardinal ligament. At this point the ureter was transected sharply with Potts scissors. The right pelvic side-wall was further dissected using clip-and-cut technique. The hypergastric artery was isolated and the anterior division was dissected free. The posterior division of the hypergastric artery was left in site. The anterior division was clamped and severed. Hemostasis on this artery was obtained by _____ (two ties of double 0 silk plus one metallic clip). Dissection was further carried down through the web and the vein returning beneath the artery was carefully identified, dissected out and ligated in a fashion similar to the artery above. Additional clips using a double side-wall clip and medial specimen single clip approach and cutting between them with the scissors was used to carry dissection all the way down to the levator muscles. The anterior lateral attachments of the bladder behind the symphysis were lysed with sharp dissection, bleeding was controlled with electrocautery. Dissection was carried down anteriorly to the level of the urethra.

Prior to all of this dissection the infundibulopelvic ligaments bilaterally had been clamped, divided and double ligated with _____ (0 chromic) sutures. The surgical specimen now consisted of uterus, tubes, ovaries, parametrium, paracolpium, vagina and bladder. All of this was placed on the vertical upward traction and in the floor of the pelvis a sharp transverse incision went through the urethra and the lower third of the vagina, thus bringing the surgical specimen, which was handed off of the field. This was subsequently carried by the surgeon to the pathologist for proper orientation for permanent cuts.

The vagina was run with continuous _____ (0 chromic)

incorporating some of the bleeding levator musculature. Additional hemostasis was obtained with electrocautery, as need be. The vaginal stump was then closed. The urethra was oversewn. The bleeders in the muscle bed were also oversewn and were electrocoagulated, as need be. The entire pelvic cavity defect was then copiously irrigated with saline solution. There was no continued bleeding.

As mentioned above, an aortic dissection had been accomplished prior to deciding to resect and that was done by simply resecting the ureters away from the aorta and vena cava and dissecting the pre-caval lymph nodes and the lymph nodes to the left of the lower abdominal aorta and submitting them for frozen section using a clip-and-cut technique.

Attention, at this time now, after resection of the anterior pelvis was directed at dissection off of the common iliac lymph node chains bilaterally, the external iliac lymph node chains bilaterally and the obturator lymph chains bilaterally. All of this was accomplished with sharp dissection using a clip-and-cut technique in the standard fashion. None of these nodes appeared to be involved with metastatic deposits, either at the time of dissection or at the prior time of palpation for anterior resection. Jackson-Pratt drains were placed in both sides of the pelvis and brought out through anterior abdominal stab wounds where they were fixed with _____ (1-0 silk) suture. An appropriate segment of ileum was then selected approximately _____ (8 cm) from the ileocecal valve and extending along for a segment length of approximately _____ (9 cm). Intraoperative pulse Doppler was used to confirm a satisfactory arterial arcade to this segment. GIAs were fired proximal and distally to the segment selected for ileoconduit formation. It is noted that, throughout the procedure, there was a good flow of urine noted through the cut ureters. An area for an ileal loop urostomy was selected in the right lower quadrant and a skin ellipse was removed. Dissection was carried down through the anterior abdominal wall. The distal end of the ileal loop was brought out through this, was opened with sharp dissections and was formed into a rose–bud formation using a triple point fixation method using _____ (0 chromic) suture. The proposed conduit was then irrigated with Betadine. The proximal end of the conduit was intact. The ureters were then trimmed, cleaned and splayed. The ureteral ileal anastomoses were then performed using _____ (4-0 GU chromic) on the splayed ureters on the ileal loop over stents. Retrograde injection of dilute Betadine solution showed that the anastomoses were water-tight. Additional fatty tissue in the area was brought in to reinforce these anastomoses and the proximal end of the ileal loop was fixed down to the mesentery with several interrupted _____ (0 chromic) sutures. Everything was then thoroughly irrigated in the abdomen and pelvis and the bowel were returned to as anatomic position as possible. The previously described peritoneal flap was used to help reperitonealize the floor of the pelvis. Sponge, instruments and needles were removed and these counts were reported as correct times two. Intravenously injected indigo carmine followed by a bolus of fluid and Lasix was seen to have egress at the end of the urinary diversion. There was no leak at the anastomotic sites.

The anterior abdominal wall was closed with a modified Smead-Jones technique using figure-of-eight sutures of _____ (1-0 Prolene). The subcutaneous tissues were irrigated copiously with saline, Betadine and saline and the skin edges were approximated with metallic clips. The sponge, instrument, count again was reported as correct. The patient was transferred to the recovery room in satisfactory condition.

Acknowledgement

This transcription was contributed by Dr Vernon Jobson then reviewed and edited by Dr John E. Turrentine.

TOTAL PELVIC EXENTERATION

Examination under anesthesia; exploratory laparotomy; periaortic lymphnode biopsies; including a low anterior colon resection with primary anastomosis & LOOP colostomy; formation of ileo-urinary conduit & sigmoid colon neovagina are included in this transcription for completeness.

Technique

The patient was brought to the operating room and intermittent venous calf compression boots were placed. Pulses were full and general anesthesia was induced. She was prepped in the usual manner for abdominal surgery and sterile draped. The abdomen was entered through a midline incision, carried in the midline just above the umbilicus. Exploration took place upon entering the abdomen. Please see author's notes. Self-retaining retractor was placed. Bowels were packed away superiorly. Attention was turned to the periaortic area and lymphnodes were sent for frozen section using a clip-and-cut technique. Frozen section returned benign.

Attention was turned anteriorly and the dissection carried down in the space of Retzius all the way to the level of the urethra. Pelvic sidewall space, specifically paravesical, perirectal spaces were joined with the dissection of the space of Retzius. Sequentially and bilaterally the vascular structures were encountered and the paravesical and perirectal spaces were clamped, cut, and ligated with interrupted sutures all the way down to the pelvic floor. The distal ureters at this point were transected with Metzenbaum scissors and tagged with triple suture for later use. Additional dissection was carried down such that the specimen was fully mobilized from the six pelvic floor spaces including the space of Retzius, space of Toldt, the paravesical spaces bilaterally and the perirectal spaces bilaterally. Surgical specimen was placed on upward traction with the only two structures holding the specimen and the patient being the distal rectum and distal vaginal attachments. The vagina was then opened with sharp dissection and cut circumferentially. Circumferential running locking stitch was placed in the distal vaginal margin to control hemostasis. Small amount of dissection was then carried cephalad up the rectovaginal septum, thus leaving a small margin of distal rectum and the rectal sphincter intact. The rectum at this point was then transected and the operative specimen passed from the table.

Irrigation was performed in the pelvis. Hemostasis was achieved with electrocautery. When the space was judged to be with good hemostasis the pelvic floor was then packed with hot, moist lap pads.

Attention was then turned to the more proximal colon, specifically the point of transection at the rectosigmoid. The descending colon was further mobilized up the splenic flexure, thus bringing the distal colon with adequate length down to the lower portions of the pelvis. It was judged at this point that the colon was adequate in length to create both a neovagina and primary anastomosis of the colon with loop colostomy.

First the approximate _____ (12–15 cm) of distal rectosigmoid colon was transected by perforating the mesentery and crossclamping and dividing with the GIA stapling device. The mesentery was kept intact and this would later form the neovagina. The more proximal sigmoid colon was mobilized and brought down to the level of the distal rectal stump. The GIA staples were removed and primary anastomosis of the colon was performed using an end-to-end anastomosis. The mucosa was anastomosed using a running stitch circumferentially. Additional seromuscular sutures were placed circumferentially using interrupted simple silk sutures of _____ (000 silk). The anastomosis was palpated through the rectum and found to be intact with adequate lumen and without leakage. The previously mentioned distal sigmoid colon segment was now brought to rest above the low anterior colon anastomosis at the level of the vagina. The GIA staples were removed and a primary anastomosis of the sigmoid colon to the vagina was made with first a running stitch of _____ (000 chromic) sewing mucosa to mucosa, followed by seromuscular sutures of approximating the bowel to distal vagina using _____ (000 silk). Again palpation of both the rectum and the vagina showed that the rectal anastomosis was not compromised and had been further reinforced by this viable colon placed above the primary anastomosis. Mesenteric blood supply was judged to be intact on both structures. Irrigation was utilized in the operative field.

In the left midquadrant of the abdomen, skin incision was made circumferentially thus creating the site for the loop colostomy. A loop of descending colon was brought through the stoma and the mesentery was perforated and a Hollister bridge was placed to stabilize this loop. It was further sutured to the skin with _____ (0 chromic) suture.

Some of the small bowel packs were removed and the distal ileum was visualized and a segment of distal ileum with a rainbow arterial arcade identified. Approximately _____ (12 cm segment) of ileum was selected and isolated at both ends with the GIA stapling device. In a converging, fan-shaped fashion, the pedicles were created in the ileo-mesentery so as to make a suitable immobile segment of ileum for construction of the urinary conduit. The distal and proximal ends of the resected ileum were then reanastomosed with a side-to-side, functional end-to-end GIA TA-35 anastomosis with staplers. The mesenteric defect was closed such that the conduit was placed below to reanastomose bowels. A circular incision was made in the right side of the abdomen and ileal stoma and was brought out through the stoma skin site. The ileal segment was found to be of adequate length. It was opened, the distal end with sharp dissection and a rosebud formation was created thus securing the ileum to the skin. The conduit was then irrigated with _____ (a saline and Betadine mixture). The course of the distal ureters was identified. These were brought through the mesentery so that they could be attached to the ileal segment. Clamps were placed in a retrograde fashion through the ileostomy down the bowel and then sharp dissection was used to create small openings in the bowel such that the ureters could be anastomosed to the ileum. Anastomosis took place using multiple simple sutures of _____ (4-0 chromic) suture. Prior to closure of the ureteral ileal anastomotic sites, single J ureteral catheters were placed in a retrograde fashion up both ureters. The anastomotic site was oversewn and reinforced with an omental patch. Reflux of Betadine into the conduit showed the anastomosis was water-tight. The base of the conduit was further secured with a few interrupted simple _____ (0 chromic) sutures to the pelvic sidewall and floor. Additional omentum was now brought in to further secure the conduit and fill the pelvis and pelvic floors as much as possible.

_____ (Jackson-Pratt) drains were placed in the pelvis and brought out through separate stab incisions in the lower abdomen and the cecum was further mobilized and brought down to the pelvis to further close the pelvic floor defect. Packs and retractors were removed. The small bowel was replaced in anatomical position as much as could be possibly done. Sponge, needle, and instrument counts were judged to be correct. The anterior abdominal wall was closed with multiple interrupted _____ (Prolene) sutures using _____ (Smead-Jones) closure technique. Subcutaneous tissue was irrigated with copious amounts of saline followed by Betadine, followed by saline. Hemostasis was judged to be intact. The skin was approximated with skin clips. Dry dressing was placed on the wound. The urinary device was placed on the urinary stoma and clear urine was noted to be coming forth. A vaseline gauze was placed over the loop colostomy. The patient was considered to be stable throughout the entire procedure and was taken to the recovery room in stable condition. She will be cared for in the intensive care unit postoperatively.

Author's notes

It is very important to transcribe indications and findings during dictation but especially crucial in cases as this – therefore samples are included below.

Sample

Indications

This patient has biopsy proven recurrent squamous cell cancer of the cervix. She has been given preoperative external beam radiation therapy and now is brought to the operating room for definitive resection with curative intent.

Findings – At the time of surgery opening of the paravesical and perirectal spaces to the pelvic floor failed to reveal any disease outside of the central recurrence. Periaortic lymphnode biopsies were performed and frozen section was benign. The upper abdomen was totally negative including right and left hemidiaphragm, right and left kidney, stomach, and small bowel. At the end of the procedure the specimen was hand carried to pathology and oriented for the pathologist so that appropriate specimen orientation would assist us postoperatively and offer some prognostic indication.

Acknowledgement

This transcription was contributed by Dr Charles H. Pippitt then reviewed and edited by Dr John E. Turrentine.

Fractional dilatation and curettage

Technique

Patient was placed on the operating table in the lithotomy position. Careful pelvic examination was performed to locate the position of the uterine corpus. The vagina and the peritoneum were cleaned with _____.

A weighted speculum was placed in the vagina. The cervix was grasped with tenaculum and gently drawn toward the vaginal outlet. A _____ (small, Gusberg, Kervorkian) curette was utilized to obtain endocervical curettings. These were obtained on Telfa pad and handed off to be sent to pathology.

A sound was then passed through the cervical canal into the uterine cavity. This was done carefully to avoid creating a false passage. Once the position of the uterus, the length of the uterine cavity (describe length), angulation between the cervical canal and uterine cavity had been ascertained, the sound was removed and the cervical canal was dilated with a small dilator. After a 3 mm dilator was passed, successively larger ones were used. After dilatation of (usually 9 mm) was reached, the dilatation was discontinued. A gauze was placed into the posterior vaginal fornix along with posterior weighted speculum retractor with a Telfa pad on top of the sponge so that blood and endometrium removed from the uterus would fall onto it.

The uterine cavity was explored initially in search of any endometrial polyps with the polyp forceps. The forceps were moved systematically across the dome of the uterus and the anterior and posterior walls. The procedure was repeated several times and then the curettage was performed with a sharp curette. This was performed in a systematic manner in which the entire area of the endometrial cavity was covered. The procedure utilizing the polyp forceps was again repeated several times after the uterine wall had been curetted to make certain that there was no area of endometrial cavity that polyp or pathology might have been missed. A malleable, bluntly serrated curette was then introduced again into the uterus and in a systematic manner the entire uterine cavity was curetted. Anterior, lateral and posterior walls were scraped gently but firmly and finally the top of the cavity was scraped with a side to side movement. After appropriate endometrial curettings had been obtained, these were placed immediately in fixative, being careful not to mash or scrape the specimens. There was no fatty tissue or unusual tissue noted. Hemostasis was judged to be excellent and all instrumentation was removed from the vagina and the patient was removed to the Recovery Room in good condition.

Groin and inguinal node dissection

Technique

The femoral canal was dissected in a manner that allowed the tissue to be removed from the surrounding artery and vein. Cloquet's nodes (nodes of Rosenmuller) were located at the femoral ring beneath the inguinal ligament. They were dissected with Metzenbaum scissors and sent for frozen section. (If these are negative for any metastatic disease, the dissection for vulvar disease can be considered complete.)

The deep inguinal chain was dissected by opening the inguinal canal from the external inguinal ring. The round ligament that passes into the caval from the peritoneal cavity (where the inguinal ring begins) was excised and the deep inguinal lymphatic tissue was removed.

The extraperitoneal pelvic lymphadenectomy was initiated by opening the external oblique muscle 2 cm above the inguinal ligament. The incision was extended as far laterally as necessary for exposure through the internal oblique and transversalis muscles. The iliac vessels were exposed by retracting the peritoneum medially.

The external iliac, common iliac, and upper portion of hypogastric vessels were included in the dissection as the entire obturator space was thoroughly cleaned. The inferior epigastric artery and vein were ligated with 2-0 _____ (silk) suture. This was performed at the point where these vessels originated from the external iliac vessels, just inside the inguinal ligament, as they coursed upward to supply the abdominal wall. The ureter was displaced medially with the parietal peritoneum so as to avoid injury during the dissection.

Following dissection of necessary nodes, a _____ (Jackson-Pratt) closed-suction drain was placed in the retro-peritoneal space as separate stab wounds were made in the abdomen for adequate removal of fluid and blood.

The inguinal canal was obliterated by closing the oblique and transversalis muscles in two-layers using a #1 _____ (delayed absorbable) suture in a "vest-over-pants" closure.

The inguinal incision was closed without tension with _____ suture and the groin specimen was sent to Pathology.

Author's notes

Transposition of the sartorius muscle is not described here as prophylactic antibiotics have essentially eliminated the need for this portion of the operation in regards to radical vulvectomy.

Hymenectomy

Technique

The patient was placed in the lithotomy position and after adequate anesthesia, she was prepped and draped in the routine manner. The _____ (partially or fully) imperforate hymen was incised at 2, 4, 8, and 10 o'clock in a stellate fashion. The individual quadrants were then excised along the lateral wall of the vagina being careful to avoid too close an excision to the vagina. The mucosal margins were reapproximated with fine 4-0 _____ (delayed absorbable) suture. Hemostasis and the result were excellent.

Author's note

Transcribe whether hematocolpos has already developed. Avoid D&C if hematocolpos has developed because of increased risk of perforating the thin overstretched uterine wall. Nothing more is needed unless the uterine mass does not regress within a few weeks. Dilatation may be needed if drainage from the uterus is unsatisfactory.

Hypogastric artery ligation

Author's notes

Transcribe why specific bleeding source was not found and/or the technical difficulty encountered in controlling hemorrhage during whatever difficult operative dissection was being performed then transcribe the following.

Technique

The peritoneum was opened on the lateral side of the common iliac artery near its bifurcation. The ureter was left attached to the medial peritoneal reflection so as to avoid disturbing its blood supply.

The posterior branch of the hypogastric artery was clearly identified then the anterior division was dissected and mobilized free from the adjacent vein. Long vascular forceps and long vascular instruments were used for dissection. #0 _____ (silk) was passed around the artery with a (an) _____ (Right angle or Adson clamp) and free-tied onto the artery. A second free-tie was placed distal to the initial ligature in similar fashion.

Important points

Remember during obstetrical procedures that involve massive hemorrhage that the ovarian artery needs to be located above the pelvic brim because of the collateral blood supply. This artery also needs to be ligated but dissected free of the ovarian vein. A hemoclip is usually all that is necessary.

Hysterectomy

Important points

- Pre-op diagnosis:

  (1) If for DUB – make certain to transcribe if the bleeding is recurrent, severe, and unresponsive to HRT and curettage (how many times?)

  (2) Adenomyosis should be rarely if ever used as a pre-op diagnosis.

  (3) Vaginal relaxation, prolapse, uterine descensus with or without SUI can be documented better if transcribed that ERT and Kegel exercises have failed or the patient is symptomatic.

  (4) Leiomyoma as a pre-op diagnosis can be enhanced by describing symptomatology (menorrhagia, metrorrhagia, discomfort, etc.) Large size (greater than 12 cm) certainly provides better description and indication for hysterectomy.

  (5) PID, Endometriosis, and other reasons for hysterectomy can be further documented if reasons why more conservative therapies were not an option or if these were tried then transcribe it!

- Location of ureters: If an IVP is done prior to surgery secondary to suspected mass effect or distortion, transcribe results during op report while locating the ureter.

- Antibiotics: Infection is the most common complication of hysterectomy. Often, the prophylactic antibiotic that is given can be included in documentation of the op report. This demonstrates that the physician not only ordered it but also checked to see that it was given.

- Choice of hysterectomy: Because of the advantages of vaginal hysterectomy over abdominal hysterectomy, if indicated and possible, the vaginal route should be the procedure of choice. LAVH is certainly a new option that can be considered somewhere in between these two choices if necessary and possible.

- EUA: Pelvic exam under anesthesia is often very helpful.

Routine use and documentation of this manuever cannot be overstated especially when correlating operative findings with pelvic exam.

- Do not use excessive force to dissect the bladder flap away from the uterus or cervix – this can cause unnecessary blood loss or inadvertent entry into the bladder.

- "WATER UNDER THE BRIDGE": Always palpate the ureters prior to clamping the uterine vessels to make certain that these are not displaced by pathology. This is a very dangerous area for possible injury to the ureters.

- Keep clamps and cutting near the uterus in an almost "rolling off" motion to avoid injury to lateral structures.

- Suspend the vaginal vault by incorporation of the round, broad, uterosacral ligaments and vaginal wall to prevent future prolapse!

- Make sure the ovaries are retained against the pelvic sidewalls and not adjacent to the vaginal cuff or the patient may subsequently complain of painful intercourse!

- If there is any doubt in regards to the integrity of the ureters, before the incision is closed, inject 5 cc of indigo carmine. Fill the bladder with approximately 200 cc of clear sterile saline and observe the ureteral orifices via cystoscopy. Within 3–5 minutes, the blue dye will be seen spurting from each orifice. (This can be performed routinely and easily if the hysterectomy is performed with the patient in Allen Universal stirrups as described in the seventh edition of TeLinde's *Operative Gynecology*.)

TOTAL ABDOMINAL HYSTERECTOMY

Technique

After satisfactory general anesthesia was obtained, an indwelling urethral catheter was placed and a careful pelvic examination under anesthesia was performed including the bimanual rectovaginal abdominal examination. Thorough Betadine vaginal preparation with particular emphasis on intravaginal cleansing of the vaginal fornices and also an abdominal prep was performed. Following the routine prep and drape, a _____ (type of incision) was carried out. This incision was carried down through the subcutaneous fascia, bringing about hemostasis with hemostats and electrocautery. Free ties were used as necessary. The fascia was entered with the scalpel blade and extended with Mayo scissors. The underlying rectus fascia and muscle layer were separated in the midline and the peritoneum was entered with two hemostats and scapel blade. The peritoneum was extended with Metzenbaum scissors and following thorough washing of the powdered gloves with normal saline and standing on the patient's right side, the right hand was placed into the upper abdomen. After appropriate washings were obtained, the right kidney, liver, gallbladder, pancreas, stomach, left kidney and para-aortic lymph nodes were palpated in sequence. (Findings are described.)

The _____ (O'Connor/O'Sullivan or Balfour) self retaining retractor was placed into the abdominal cavity and opened for pelvic exposure. Adhesions were released so that the intestines could be placed in the upper abdomen and held there with _____ (wet lap packs or GYN bag).

The patient was placed in a modest Trendelenburg position and the round ligaments were bilaterally grasped with Kelly clamps near the uterine cornu, cut and ligated with a 0-_____ (delayed absorbable) suture. The sutures were tagged bilaterally with a hemostat and left long.

The anterior leaves of the broad ligaments were incised to the point of reflection of the bladder peritoneum on the uterus. The avascular areas of the broad ligaments were located, incised, and the fallopian tubes and ovarian ligaments (infundibulo-pelvic ligaments if BSO to be performed) were triply clamped as close as possible to the uterine corpus. Free ties using 0-_____ (delayed absorbable) sutures were placed as the second clamp of each cut pedicle bilaterally was removed. A 0-_____ (delayed absorbable) suture was placed in front of each of the first ligatures in the center of the pedicles beneath the remaining clamps and passing the free ends of the suture around the tips and heels of each clamp prior to tying. Both clamps were then removed.

The midline reflection of the bladder peritoneum on to the uterus was then freed by extending the incision in to the anterior leaf of the broad ligament. The bladder was separated from the lower uterine segment and upper cervix by careful sharp dissection with the fascial fibers beneath the bladder wall. Mobilization of the bladder away from the cervix and upper anterior vaginal wall was performed. The posterior leaf of the broad ligament was then cut on either side parallel with the lateral side of the uterus down to the point of origin on the uterosacral ligaments behind the cervix. Incising the anterior and posterior broad ligament peritoneum allowed the uterine vessels to be exposed and skeletonized with the Metzenbaum scissors bilaterally.

At this point the lower portion of the pelvic ureters were palpated as they coursed beneath the uterine arteries bilaterally, lateral to the internal cervical os bilaterally, and passed medially through the base of the broad ligament to enter the trigone of the bladder. With wide mobilization and displacement of the bladder base from the cervix, and with traction on the uterine corpus, the ureters were located lateral and inferior to the point of clamping of the uterine vessels. After completely exposing the uterine vessels by completely skeletonizing these vessels, they were then triply clamped bilaterally with curved _____ (Ochsner or Kocher) clamps. As the lowest clamp was placed initially, it was placed at the level of the internal cervical os and then also at right angles to the lower uterine segment. The other two clamps were placed above this first clamp. This was performed bilaterally. The vessels were cut with a scalpel between the upper and middle clamps and freed from the uterus by extending the incision around the tip of the middle clamp. Care was taken to avoid incising the tissue beyond the tip of the lowest clamp. Sutures were placed precisely in the angle of the incision and at the tip of the clamp, making certain that all vessels and the clamps were secured by ligature. This was performed bilaterally. The uterine vessels were doubly ligated with 0-_____ (delayed absorbable) suture with ligation of the tissue within the lowest clamp initially. As the first suture was tied bilaterally, the clamps were removed. As the second ligatures were placed and tied, the middle clamps were removed bilaterally. Following bilateral ligation of the uterine vessels, straight _____ (Ochsner or Ballentine) clamps were placed between the uterine vessels and bilateral sides of the uterus. The tissue was clamped bilaterally in the uppermost parts of the cardinal ligaments. This was then cut and suture ligated with 0-_____ (delayed absorbable) sutures. The uterus was pulled forward and upward to expose and stress the uterosacral ligaments posteriorly.

Each uterosacral ligament was clamped with a _____ (curved Ochsner or Ballentine clamp). Particular care was taken to avoid the pelvic portion of the ureter as it coursed along the base of the broad ligament. The uterosacral ligaments were then clamped, incised, and ligated with 0-_____ (delayed absorbable) sutures. Continued blunt and sharp dissection inferiorly in the center of the cul-de-sac between the ligated uterosacral ligaments developed a plane between the cervix and the vagina anteriorly and the anterior rectal wall posteriorly. At this point dissection of the bladder base away from the anterior vaginal wall was completed.

With the uterus under firm traction, the thumb and index finger from the same hand was made readily opposed below the cervix and further dissection of the base of the bladder anterior and the rectum posteriorly was accomplished. Particular attention to the pubovesicocervical fascia was then given as a small incision was made in the fascia anterior to the cervix just below the level of the internal cervical os and the ligated uterine vessels. As the edges of the fascia were retracted laterally a pale avascular area of the anterior surface of the cervix and the vagina could be seen. The blunt end of scalpel was used in dissecting the loosened fibers of the pubovesicocervical fascia from the cervix. Dissection was continued with a sponge forcep until the fascia had been reflected far laterally off the anterior surface of the cervix and upper vagina. The whitish fascial plane of the vagina came into view. Dissection of the remaining portion of the cardinal ligaments were carried out by placing _____ (straight Ochsner or Ballentine) clamps inside the cut edges of the pubovesicocervical fascia. The lateral vaginal fornix was identified. The anterior and posterior walls of the vagina were clamped together at each lateral vaginal angle using a (an) _____ (Ochsner or Ballentine) clamp.

The uterus was removed by _____ [a circumferential incision made into the vagina as close to the cervix as possible using the curved _____ (Jorgenson) scissors] or a _____ (#170 or #200) polyroticulator was placed carefully under the cervix, clamped, and locked into place. The cervix was cut away from the vaginal cuff with the _____ (Jorgenson) scissors above the locked clamp. The polyroticulator was then unlocked and removed with absorbable staples demonstrating good placement and good hemostasis. The entire cervix was removed with the uterine corpus.

(If roticulator is not used, transcribe paragraph similar to this.)
_____ (Ochsner or Ballentine) clamps on the bilateral vaginal angles were replaced with transfixion Richardson sutures on each angle. The free margin of the vagina was then reefed with a continuous interlocking suture of 2-0 _____ (delayed absorbable) suture. (If a drain is being placed through to the vagina, now is the time to transcribe it.*) Hemostasis was maintained with figure of eight sutures utilizing 2-0 _____ (delayed absorbable) suture in the vaginal vault.

Posterior and anterior culdoplasty was then performed. The right round ligament was then located and with the suture that had been placed on the round ligament, this hemostat was removed, and the suture was brought down into the vaginal corner suture. It was tied into place along with the suture from the cardinal ligament which had been left in place. These were reapproximated together. The same was performed on the left side as on the right side. Additional suspension of the vaginal vault was combined with peritonealization suture. In this technique use of a continuous 0-_____ (delayed absorbable) suture was used to pierce the vaginal wall and it was passed through the ligated pedicle of the angle of the vagina and the free margin of the cardinal ligament, staying distal to the original cardinal ligament ligature. The suture was then passed through the anterior bladder peritoneum near the round ligament, and then continued through the free margin of the round ligament and the remaining edge of the anterior leaf of the broad ligament incorporating the free margin of the utero-ovarian ligament and continued posteriorly along the cut edge of the posterior leaf of the broad ligament incorporating the uterosacral ligament. This suture finally pierced the posterior edge of the vaginal wall near the midline. The ligatures were all tied firmly in the midline. The same was performed on the left side as was performed on the right and this accomplished vaginal vault suspension and peritonealization on each side. The tip of the broad ligament was closed separately with a purse string suture of 3-0 _____ (delayed absorbable) suture and the free margin of the pedicle was buried beneath the peritoneum allowing the ovaries to be retàined high against the pelvic wall and not anchored to the vaginal vault. This was performed bilaterally.

Peritonealization was completed by suturing the bladder peritoneum to the cul-de-sac peritoneum with 3-0 _____ (delayed absorbable) suture. This suture was initiated near the angle of the vagina where the anterior peritoneum was pierced and the peritoneum over the round ligament and infundibulopelvic ligament was picked up before the cul-de-sac peritoneum was sutured. The suture was tied and then continued to the opposite angle of the vagina as a continuous suture approximating the bladder and cul-de-sac peritoneum. The pelvis was inspected and thoroughly irrigated with normal saline solution. The normal saline was suctioned off with the suction tip and the lap pads and self retaining retractor were removed.

The peritoneum was closed in a continuous fashion utilizing 2-0 _____ in a 3 point stitch to avert the cut peritoneal edges and to make intraperitoneal suture line as smooth as possible. Hemostasis was judged to be excellent and the muscles were reapproximated in the midline with interrupted sutures of 2-0 _____. The fascial edges were approximated with single #1 _____ suture utilizing a modification of the far/near, near/far, suture method. Subcutaneous fat was approximated with interrupted sutures of 3-0 _____ suture following thorough irrigation of this area. Skin closure was then performed and following cleansing of the skin a (Telfa and bandage) were applied with routine dressing. Instrument , lap and sponge counts were all correct. The patient was removed to the Recovery Room in stable condition.

Author's notes

*If a polyroticulator was *not* used, transcribe. If a roticulator was used, omit paragraph 10. If a drain was placed through to the vagina, it must be described.

TOTAL ABDOMINAL HYSTERECTOMY WITH BILATERAL SALPINGO-OOPHORECTOMY (BRIEF FORM STYLE)

Technique

The patient was prepped and draped in the usual manner with the legs placed in Universal Allen stirrups. Examination under anesthesia was performed under sterile conditions following thorough Betadine prep. A Foley catheter was placed into the urethral orifice until urine was obtained and the catheter was left in place. The surgical prep and drape was completed and then gloves and gown were changed. A lower abdominal transverse Maylard incision was performed and carried down through the subcutaneous tissue to the fascia. Hemostasis was performed using hemostats and electrocautery. The fascia was entered with scalpel blade and extended with Mayo scissors. The underlying rectus fascia and muscle layer was separated in the midline and the peritoneum was entered with two hemostats and Metzenbaum scissors. The incision was extended with Metzenbaum scissors following washing of the gloves in the splash basin. Standing on the patient's right side, the abdominal and peritoneal washings were obtained with catheter. The upper abdomen was explored, including the right liver, kidney, gall bladder, pancreas, stomach, left kidney, and periaortic lymph nodes. The findings were normal. The Bookwalter self-retaining retractor was placed into the abdomen with lap-packs to provide adequate exposure.

Round ligaments were bilaterally clamped, cut, and suture-ligated using curved Ochsner clamps and _____ (#2-0, delayed absorbable) suture. The anterior leaves of the broad ligaments were then entered to the point of reflection on the bladder and the avascular portion of the broad ligament was incised with scissors, thus making a window in the broad ligament bilaterally. After fully assessing the condition of the ovaries, it was decided that bilateral salpingo-oophorectomy would be in the best interest of this patient. Infundibulopelvic ligaments were bilaterally triply clamped, cut, and suture-ligated with both a free-tie and a suture ligature. The uterine vessels were exposed and the lower portion of the pelvic ureters were palpated as each coursed beneath the uterine arteries bilaterally, lateral to the internal cervical os bilaterally, passing medially through the base of the broad ligament until each entered the trigone of the bladder. With wide mobilization, displacement of the bladder base from the cervix using a sponge stick and with traction on the uterine corpus, the ureters were located lateral and inferior to the point of clamping the uterine vessels. The uterine vessels were triply clamped bilaterally with curved Ochsner clamps. The clamps had been placed at the level of the internal cervical os at right angles to the lower uterine segment. The other two clamps were placed above the first clamp. This was performed bilaterally.

The uterine vessels were cut with scalpel blade between the upper and middle clamps and freed from the uterus by extending the incision around the tip of the middle clamp. Care was taken to avoid incising the tissue beyond the tip of the lowest clamp. The sutures were placed precisely at an angle of the incision and at the tip of the clamp making certain that all vessels and clamp were secured by ligature. This was performed bilaterally.

The uterine vessels were then doubly ligated with _____ (0-delayed absorbable) suture bilaterally. The clamps were removed and then straight Ballentine clamps were placed between the uterine vessels and the ligated uterine vessels dropped laterally away from the uterus bilaterally. The cardinal ligaments were bilaterally clamped and suture-ligated with _____ (0-delayed absorbable) suture. Ballentine clamps were used to perform further isolation of the uterosacral ligaments, as these were clamped, cut, and suture-ligated with _____ (0-delayed absorbable) suture bilaterally. Further clamping, cutting, and suture-ligating of the uterosacral ligaments on the bilateral sides of the uterus was performed, taking care to avoid the pelvic portions of the ureters, as each coursed along the base of the broad ligament.

The bladder base was dissected away from the anterior vaginal wall, using both sharp and blunt dissection. With the uterus under firm traction and the thumb and index finger from the same hand made readily opposed below the cervix, further dissection was performed along the base of the bladder anterior and posterior along the rectum. Particular attention to the pubovesicocervical fascia was made as the _____ (#170 polyreticulator) was placed under the cervix. The reticulator was applied and staples clamped into place. As the reticulator was locked and staples applied, the Jorgenson scissors were then used to dissect the cervix away from the vaginal cuff. The entire cervix was removed from the operative field and then entire uterus, cervix, and bilateral ovaries and tubes were sent to pathology.

Sutures on the round ligaments and uterosacral and cardinal ligaments were reapproximated along the corner of the vaginal cuff to provide support to the new pelvic floor. The peritoneum was then closed over the bladder cuff with _____ (2-0 delayed absorbable) suture. The entire area was irrigated thoroughly prior to closing the bladder cuff and hemostasis was judged to be excellent.

The peritoneum was closed with _____ (2-0 delayed absorbable) suture in a continuous fashion. The muscle layer was closed in an interrupted fashion with (0-delayed absorbable) suture. The fascia was closed with _____ (#1-delayed absorbable) suture in a continuous fashion. Each layer was irrigated thoroughly prior to closure. The subcutaneous tissue was closed with _____ (3-0 plain) suture in a continuous fashion. The skin was closed with skin staples. The incision was wiped clean with a wet lap-dry lap and bandage was applied. The patient tolerated the procedure very well.

Cystoscopy was not performed because ureters were bilaterally palpated and visualized to be intact and very functional during and after the procedure.

RADICAL HYSTERECTOMY

Exploratory laparotomy; bilateral salpingo-oophorectomy; periaortic & pelvic lymphadenectomies bilateral; lysis of adhesions are included in this transcription for completeness.

Technique

The patient was placed in modified dorsal-lithotomy position after IVCC booties had been connected, and general anesthesia had been induced. A Foley catheter was inserted. She was placed supine and after exam under anesthesia had been carried out, the findings of which are noted above, she was then prepped and draped in a sterile fashion. The abdominal cavity was opened through midline vertical incision extending from symphysis to umbilicus. On entry, exploration was carried out, findings noted above. The upper abdominal viscera were all palpated _____ (normal).

Attention was turned to the pelvis after self-retaining retractor had been placed and the bowels packed away superiorly. The uterus was grasped with large Kelly clamps bilaterally and elevated. Round ligaments were divided using _____ (an LDS CO_2 powered device). The vesicouterine reflection was sharply incised transversely. The infundibulopelvic ligaments were isolated and when the ureters were seen to be clear and free, the infundibulopelvic ligaments were divided with _____ (an LDS CO_2 powered device). Additional _____ (0 chromic ties) were placed on these pedicles. Bilaterally the perivesical and perirectal spaces were opened down to the levator muscles. The course of the distal obliterated hypogastric arteries bilaterally was identified and these vessels skeletonized, thereby they were able to be retracted laterally out of harm's way. All the pelvic and periaortic nodal areas were palpated and there was no adenopathy appreciated.

First on the right, the origin of the uterine vessels were identified, the web was carefully retracted so as to expose it satisfactorily. The ureter reflected medial out of harm's way and the structures of the web, including the uterine vessels were taken at their origin, and/or insertion into the hypogastric artery or vein respectively. All this was a clip and cut technique. It was carried out down to the level of the levator muscles. An identical procedure was repeated on the opposite side.

The course of the right ureter was identified, it was dissected off the peritoneal reflection posteriorly and was skeletonized down to its entry into the cardinal ureteric tunnel. It was unroofed using _____ (Lahey clamps). The specimen side was clamped and the patient side was tied with _____ (00 chromic). The ureter was dissected all the way down to its splaying into the bladder base. Identical procedure was repeated on the opposite side.

The rectovaginal septum was opened with sharp dissection and the rectum pushed away posteriorly. The ureterosacral ligaments bilaterally were taken near their insertion into the bony pelvic wall with _____ (Heaney clamps) using a clamp, cut, and Heaney ligature _____ (0 chromic) technique. Laterally parametrial pedicles were developed with Heaney clamps. The entire surgical specimen consisting of cervix and corpus uteri, as well as both tubes and ovaries, parametrium, paracolpos and upper one-third of the vagina was placed on additional further upward traction. The ureters were reflected laterally out of harm's way, the rectum posteriorly and the bladder anteriorly. Kidney pedicle C-clamps were placed. Below these Heaney clamps were placed and a transverse incision freed the above mentioned surgical specimen. Modified Aldridge angle sutures were placed in the lateral vaginal angles, and the posterior cuff was run in continuity to the parietal peritoneum of the colon, the anterior cuff was run in continuity with the parietal peritoneum overlying the bladder, all with _____ (0 chromic). Then a rainbow arcade stitch was placed from side-to-side thus recreating the upper one-third of the vagina. The pelvis was irrigated and hemostasis was noted to be satisfactory.

Bilateral aortic and pelvic lymphadenectomy was then accomplished from just below the level of the renal vessels down to the level of the circumflex iliac veins into the floor of the obturator fossa below the level of the obturator nerves bilaterally. Great care was taken at all times to avoid injury to the ureters, the vessels, and the nerves in the operated areas. Nodal material was labeled as to site of origin and was removed using a clip-and-cut technique. Bilaterally, drains were placed in the retroperitoneal areas, the pelvis was irrigated and hemostasis noted to be satisfactory. Exit sites of the peritoneal drains were secured on the anterior abdominal wall with box type stitches.

One amp of indigo carmine was injected along with a fluid bolus. There was a prompt clearing of the dye through the kidneys with ureters found to peristalsis normally. There was no evidence of extravasation of the blue urine from either ureter or the bladder.

Bowels returned to an anatomic position. Sponge, instrument, and needle count reported as correct times two. The abdominal wall was closed with modified Smead-Jones figure of eight _____ (#1 Prolene). The subcutaneous layer was irrigated with Betadine, and saline. Skin closure was with _____ (metallic clips). Dry, pressure dressing was placed on the wound. The patient tolerated the operative procedure well and was transferred to the recovery room in satisfactory condition.

Acknowledgement

This transcription was contributed by Dr Charles H. Pippitt, then reviewed and edited by Dr John E. Turrentine.

TOTAL VAGINAL HYSTERECTOMY (WITH SUSPENSION OF THE VAGINAL VAULT)

Technique

After the patient was anesthetized, a pelvic examination was carried out under anesthesia. (Findings may be transcribed.) After proper scrub, the patient was placed in the dorsolithotomy position with the hips located at the edge of the table so that a weighted speculum could swing free, the vulva, perineum and vagina were thoroughly washed with Betadine. The bladder was emptied with a catheter and clamped. With the cervix exposed, it was grasped with a tenaculum and pulled strongly into view. 10 ml of dilute Neo-Synephrine solution (1:200,000) was injected into the anterior and posterior vaginal fornices.

A semi lunar incision was made through the mucosa of the vaginal fornix just above the portio but below the attachment of the bladder. The bladder was freed from the anterior surface of the uterus by sharp dissection up to the plica vesicouterinea. After the loose areolar plane was entered and the fascial attachments were excised beneath the bladder with the curved Mayo scissors, the dissection was completed with the finger covered with gauze. The free peritoneal fold was identified and incised. A narrow bladed retractor was inserted into the peritoneal cavity to hold the bladder and the ureters forward. Following this entry into the anterior cul-de -sac, the cervix was pulled strongly forward and a semi lunar incision was made through the vaginal mucosa at the height of the posterior fornix and the anterior and posterior incisions were joined on each side of the cervix. Care was taken to avoid injury to the rectum. After cutting through the mucosa, the loose areolar plane was entered and the space was developed by sharp dissection until the peritoneum was visible. The cul–de-sac was explored and a narrow right angle retractor was introduced. The peritoneal reflection was then excised under direct vision. Pushing back the mucosa, the peritoneum exposed the base of the cardinal ligaments.

The base of the cardinal ligament was clamped separately by a Heaney clamp and was then cut on the uterine side and the clamp was replaced by a fixation suture using #1 _____ (delayed absorbable) suture. Next the uterosacral ligament was clamped with a Heaney clamp, excised, and transfixed with a similar suture. The ligated pedicle was held for later plication by an identifying hemostat and this would be used later during a vaginal vault suspension. The retractor was placed in both the anterior and posterior cul-de-sac to allow excellent exposure of the left broad ligament while displacing the bladder, ureter and rectum. After the base of the cardinal ligament and left uterosacral ligament were separately cut and ligated, the uterine vessels could be seen.

The vessels were similarly clamped, cut, but replaced by a nontransfixion suture using a #1 _____ (delayed absorbable) suture. In successive similar steps, the broad ligament on the left was disposed of as high as possible, picking up the anterior peritoneum above the uterine vessels with each successive pedicle.

When further progress on the left could not be made, the retractors were shifted to the right of the patient and the right cardinal ligament was clamped, cut and ligated in similar fashion. The uterosacral ligament was clamped, excised and transfixed separately and the ligature was held with a hemostat. In similar steps on the right the uterine vessels were ligated but not transfixed and the right broad ligament was severed from the uterus as high as exposure allowed. After the broad ligaments had been excised as high as possible on each side of the uterine body, the cervix was pulled superiorly.

The uterine body then presented itself at the posterior opening, where it was grasped by a Lahey clamp. This was partially pulled outside the introitus. The upper portion of the broad ligament, the uterine end of the tube, and the suspensory ligament of the ovary and the round ligament on the left side were now identified and were carefully inspected. These structures were incorporated into the cornual portion of the broad ligament, which was clamped, cut and doubly ligated. This was performed with a free tie to occlude the vascular pedicle and then it was transfixed with a stay suture placed on the outside of the previous ligature. The outer ligature on the pedicle from the tip of the broad ligament was held with a Kelly clamp to identify this ligament at the time of peritonealization and suspension of the vaginal vault. After the left side of the uterus was freed, the right cornual region was clamped, excised and ligated by similar technique.

The uterus was removed and inspected to see whether any pathological process existed and the findings can be seen as above. After the uterus was removed a small wet laparotomy pack was held by a small clamp.

Suspension of the vaginal vault was performed by a continuous suture utilizing #1 _____ (delayed absorbable) suture placed through the lateral vaginal wall and adjacent to the peritoneum. The suture was continued through the tip of the broad ligament, cardinal ligament and uterosacral ligament before returning through the vaginal wall. After suspension was completed on both sides the patient culdoplasty suture was passed through the uterosacral ligament, cul-de-sac, peritoneum, and opposite ligament which was the internal suture. The second suture was placed slightly higher. External culdoplasty sutures were placed through the posterior fornix and passed through each uterosacral ligament before returning through cul-de-sac, peritoneum, and posterior fornix. A purse string suture was used to encircle the peritoneal surface as the highest internal suture utilizing 0 _____ (delayed absorbable) suture. The peritoneal suture was placed in a manner in which the vascular pedicles were in an extraperitoneal position so as to avoid intraperitoneal bleeding.

The suspension sutures in the lateral vaginal angles were tied and the uterosacral plication sutures were now tied both internally and in the posterior fornix. The purse string suture was then tied and found to be adequately closed in that a finger could not be admitted. Transverse closure of the vaginal vault was then performed with figure of eight sutures utilizing 0 Vicryl. _____ inch iodoform packing was then placed in the vagina. Estimated blood loss was _____ . Instruments, needle, sponge, and lap counts were all correct.

TOTAL VAGINAL HYSTERECTOMY
(WITH LASH INCISION AND MORCELLATION)

Technique

After the patient was anesthetized, a pelvic examination was carried out under anesthesia. (Findings may be transcribed.) After proper scrub, the patient was placed in the dorsolithotomy position with the hips located at the edge of the table so that a weighted speculum could swing free, the vulva, perineum and vagina were thoroughly washed with _____ . The bladder was emptied with catheter and clamped. With the cervix exposed, it was grasped with a tenaculum and pulled strongly into view.

An incision around the cervix with the Bovie unit was made through the mucosa of the vaginal fornix just above the portio but below the attachment of the bladder and through the vaginal mucosa at the height of the posterior fornix. Dissection was performed until the peritoneal fold was identified then this area was incised and a narrow bladed retractor was inserted. The posterior peritoneum was then excised under direct vision and the cul-de-sac was explored and a narrow right angle retractor was introduced. Pushing back the mucosa, the peritoneum exposed the base of the cardinal ligaments.

The base of the cardinal ligaments were clamped separately by Heaney clamps, cut and replaced by fixation sutures using #1 _____ (delayed absorbable) suture. Next the uterosacral ligaments were clamped, excised, and transfixed with a similar suture. The ligated pedicles were held for later plication by identifying hemostats.

The uterine vessels were similarly clamped, cut, but replaced by nontransfixion sutures using a #1 _____ (delayed absorbable) suture. In successive similar steps, the broad ligaments bilaterally were disposed of as high as possible, picking up the anterior peritoneum above the uterine vessels with each successive pedicle.

It was noted, however, that the uterine body was too large to present itself at the introitus therefore a lash incision was carried out along both sides of the lower uterine segment in an attempt to invert the uterus. Completion of the operation using only this method was unsuccessful therefore morcellation was performed in that the cervix and lower uterine segment was amputated first followed by several other portions of myometria until there was enough exposure in order to grasp the remaining uterus with a _____ (Lahey or double or tooth tenaculum).

The remaining uterus was partially pulled outside the introitus. The upper portions of the broad ligaments, the uterine ends of the tubes and the suspensory ligaments of the ovaries and the round ligaments on the both sides were now identified and were carefully inspected. These structures were incorporated into the cornual portions of the broad ligaments, which were clamped, cut and doubly ligated. This was performed with free ties to occlude the vascular pedicles and these were transfixed with stay sutures placed on the outside of the previous ligatures. The outer ligatures on the pedicles from the tips of the broad ligaments were held with Kelly clamps to identify these ligaments at the time of peritonealization and suspension of the vaginal vault.

The uterus, having been removed in portions, was examined for gross pathology. *(Describe findings here or in pretechnique note.)* After the uterus was removed a small wet laparotomy pack was held by a small clamp.

Suspension of the vaginal vault was performed by a continuous suture utilizing #1 _____ (delayed absorbable) suture placed through the lateral vaginal wall and adjacent to the peritoneum. The suspension sutures in the lateral vaginal angles were tied and the uterosacral plication sutures were now tied both internally and in the posterior fornix. The purse string suture was then tied and found to be adequately closed in that a finger could not be admitted.

Transverse closure of the vaginal vault was then performed with figure of eight sutures utilizing 0 Vicryl. _____ inch iodoform packing was then placed in the vagina. Estimated blood loss was _____ . Instruments, needle, sponge, and lap counts were all correct.

Hysteroscopy

Important points

- Contraindications:
  IUP, PID, Invasive endometrial cancer

- Distending media
  Drawbacks:

CO$_2$
1) hypercarbia
2) acidosis
3) cardiac arrhythmias
4) cardiac arrest
5) embolization
6) death

D5W
1) low viscosity
2) low ability to
   disperse blood
   from field

32% Dextran 70 (Hyskon)
1) excessive fluid
   absorption-----
   a) hyponatermia
   b) pulmonary edema
   c) DIC
2) adherence to instruments
   can damage valves and
   optical components
3) care must be taken
   not to over dilate
   the cervix or Hyskon
   will drain too quickly
   and make distention
   difficult

- Never use laparoscopic insufflator to insufflate or distend the uterine cavity. (HysteroFlator automatically shuts off at 200 mmHg.)

HYSTEROSCOPIC ABLATION OF THE ENDOMETRIUM

Author's notes

Following transcription for diagnostic hysteroscopy which proceeded a comment in regards to pre-operative therapy such as danazol 600 mg-800 mg daily for four weeks or Synarel 7.5 mg etc... to produce atrophic and thin endometrium, the following transcription can be applied.

Technique

_____ (6–8 ml) of a dilute solution of vasopressin (10 units in 10 ml sterile saline) was injected into the cervical and paracervical areas decrease blood loss. Dilation of the cervix to _____ (9–10 mm) was performed to accommodate the operative sheath of the 26 French resectoscope. This allowed a water tight seal but with the ability to insert and withdraw the instrument. (Rollerball, rollerbarrel, or Nd-YAG laser can be used at this point but since rollerball and loop electrode is the author's preference, this is transcribed).

Uterine distension was provided by a _____ (3% surbitol, glycine, etc) solution fed into the inflow port on the sheath and collected by low suction from the outflow port. Cutting current of _____ (usually 120 W) and a coagulation current of _____ (65 W) was utilized as major _____ (lesions, myoma, etc.) were shaved with the resectoscope loop electrode to the level of the endometrium. Care was taken to avoid perforation of the myometrium. The rollerball electrode was used along the cornu and lower uterine segment using combination resection and coagulation to a depth of _____ (3–4 mm). The loop and rollerball were used interchangeably until the result was noted to be _____ (good, excellent, describe).

The procedure was then discontinued and instrumentation removed from the pelvis. The patient tolerated the procedure very well.

HYSTEROSCOPIC BALLOON TUBOPLASTY (TRANSVAGINAL FALLOPIAN TUBE RECANALIZATION)

Technique

After proximal tubal obstruction had been demonstrated by HSG and the patient had been given two days of prophylactic oral antibiotics consisting of _____ (doxycycline or Augmentin), the patient's follicular phase of her menstrual cycle was confirmed prior to beginning the procedure.

The patient was given IV _____ (Fentenyl or Versed) as needed while her vital signs were monitored by _____ (Dynamap, nurse's name, etc...). The cervix was prepped with _____ (Betadine, Hibiclens) after bivalve speculum was in proper position.

The cervix was then cannulated by means of a coaxial angiographic catheter and guide wire system consisting of a _____ (6 French) catheter and a (0.038 inch J-wire) The catheter was advanced to the ostium of the occluded tube and wedged into the ostium. Hyskon (or other radiographic material) was injected but did not clear the tubal obstruction. *(In some cases this clears the obstruction.)*

A smaller _____ (3 French) catheter with a smaller, flexible _____ (0.018 inch) guidewire was advanced in a bougie type of dilatation through the interstitial portion of the fallopian tube until recanalization could be confirmed with _____ (Hyskon or other contrast material) being noted to demonstrate a fully patent fallopian tube.

The procedure was repeated with the opposite fallopian tube as above until patency was confirmed.

DIAGNOSTIC HYSTEROSCOPY

Technique

Bimanual examination was performed to determine the size of the uterus and the orientation of the corpus in relation to the cervix. Vaginal preparation was performed using _____ (Betadine, Hibiclens) then further disinfection was performed over a wide area of the exposed cervix after the _____ (bivalve, weighted and Simons) speculum provided good exposure.

Distending media using _____ (CO_2, glycine, D5W, 32% Dextran 70) was set at a flow rate not to exceed _____ . A single-toothed tenaculum was placed on the anterior cervical lip and held with the left hand. Traction corrected for _____ (anti, retro) version. Optical assembly and end of the hysteroscope was inserted into the external cervical os. Endocervical canal was examined and found to _____ (be within normal limits or describe pathology). The plicae palmatae was readily visible.

Instrumentation was advanced until resistance was met then after _____ (10–20 seconds) the _____ (distention media) dilated the internal os enough to allow further advancement into the uterine cavity under _____ (direct, video) visualization. Flow rate was then maintained at _____ (ml/min) to allow systematic examination of the anterior, posterior, sidewalls, fundus, and cornua of the intrauterine cavity. (Describe findings.)

HYSTEROSCOPIC MYOMECTOMY

Author's notes

Assuming the patient wishes to maintain fertility, this procedure is transcribed in the following manner. Otherwise, laser ablation or cautery would be considered an option. After inspection of the uterus, describe the findings.

Technique

After distention of the uterus with _____ (D5W, sorbitol, glycine, or Dextran 70), inspection of the uterus was performed. The large pedunculated fibroid was excised by transecting its stalk with the hysteroscopic scissors and controlling minimal bleeding with the _____ (cautery or laser). A smaller pedunculated fibroid was twisted off and extracted with the hysteroscopic polyp forceps. The submucous components of the intramural fibroids that were less than 2 x 2 cm were resected by placing the resectoscopic loop behind the tumor and drawing it toward the endoscope while applying _____ (30–40) watts of cutting current. Care was taken to avoid the tubal orifices while the resectoscope was used to shave the tumor into slices. Measuring _____ (4 mm x 3 cm for example), these floated in the (sorbitol, Dextran 70, D5W, etc.). These shavings and fragments ran out, as the resectoscope was withdrawn from its sheath. The remainder of the tissue pieces were pulled out with the hysteroscopic ovum forceps. The uterus was irrigated with normal saline to remove clots, bubbles, and debris then the resectoscope was reinserted, the uterus redistended, and the operation continued in similar manner until all myomae were absent.

The patient tolerated the procedure very well. Instructions have been given to her that include two doses of prophylactic antibiotics consisting of _____ . She was also given a ten day course of _____ (po estrogen, Premarin, Ogen, Estrace) in the dose of _____ (usually 1.25 mg daily). She is to avoid coitus for _____ (3–4 weeks) and has been advised to undergo hysterogram approximately _____ (2–3) months postoperatively.

HYSTEROSCOPY FOR UTERINE SEPTAL RESECTION

Technique

After a dilute solution of _____ (sorbitol, Dextran 70, etc.) was provided through a _____ (9–10 mm) dilated cervix, the hysteroscopic scissors were used to cut central and lateral scars. *(Sometimes passing the scissors between the scope and the endocervical canal offers the greatest opportunity for free hand surgery. Transcribe whether the instrument is passed through the sheath or between the scope and endocervical canal.)* After all the adhesions had been lysed, tubal patency was checked via injection of methylene blue. Laparoscopically, the patency of the tubes appeared _____ (bilaterally adequate, only unilaterally to spill, etc.).

After tubal patency was evaluated, a _____ (Lippes Loop) was inserted to help separate the uterine walls. The patient was then placed on _____ (high-dose estrogens, Premarin 1.25 mg po qid for two 21 day courses, separated by one week of rest). The patient tolerated the procedure well and has been instructed to have the IUD removed after the end of her two treatment periods and then undergo another hysterosalpingography.

Author's notes

Diagnostic hysteroscopy is first transcribed and usually this is also performed in conjunction with laparoscopy since perforation is considered to occur most often in hysteroscopic surgery for Asherman's Syndrome. Laparoscopy can be transcribed here also. 'Solos' offers a dual camera system which is excellent for performing laparoscopy and hysteroscopy simultaneously.

If significant bleeding occurs, a Silastic rubber balloon can be used as a tamponade by inflating it for several hours then reducing the pressure and leaving it in place for up to one week.

Inguinal and groin node dissection

Technique

The femoral canal was dissected in a manner that allowed the tissue to be removed from the surrounding artery and vein. Cloquet's nodes (nodes of Rosenmuller) were located at the femoral ring beneath the inguinal ligament. They were dissected with Metzenbaum scissors and sent for frozen section. *(If these are negative for any metastatic disease, the dissection for vulvar disease can be considered complete.)*

The deep inguinal chain was dissected by opening the inguinal canal from the external inguinal ring. The round ligament that passes into the canal from the peritoneal cavity (where the inguinal ring begins) was excised and the deep inguinal lymphatic tissue was removed.

The extraperitoneal pelvic lymphadenectomy was initiated by opening the external oblique muscle 2 cm above the inguinal ligament. The incision was extended as far laterally as necessary for exposure through the internal oblique and transversalis muscles. The iliac vessels were exposed by retracting the peritoneum medially.

The external iliac, common iliac, and upper portion of hypogastric vessels were included in the dissection as the entire obtorator space was thoroughly cleaned. The inferior epigastric artery and vein were ligated with 2-0 _____ (silk) suture. This was performed at the point where these vessels originated from the external iliac vessels, just inside the inguinal ligament, as they coursed upward to supply the abdominal wall. The ureter was displaced medially with the parietal peritoneum so as to avoid injury during the dissection.

Following dissection of necessary nodes, a _____ (Jackson-Pratt) closed-suction drain was placed in the retro-peritoneal space as separate stab wounds were made in the abdomen for adequate removal of fluid and blood.

The inguinal canal was obliterated by closing the oblique and transversalis muscles in two-layers using a #1 _____ (delayed absorbable) suture in a "vest-over-pants" closure. The inguinal incision was closed without tension with suture and the groin specimen was sent to pathology.

Author's notes

If Cloquet's nodes are negative for any metastatic disease, the dissection for vulvar disease can be considered complete.

Transpostion of the sartorius muscle is not described here as prophylactic antibiotics have essentially eliminated the need for this portion of the operation in regards to radical vulvectomy.

Laparoscopy

Overview

Operative laparoscopy can include operative laparoscopy with chromotubation, laser laparoscopy, videolaserlaparoscopy, and innumerable other laparoscopic procedures other than diagnostic laparoscopy.

Most laparoscopic procedures, however, begin with basic steps in preparation for the operative portion of the laparoscopy. It is sometimes during this initial preparation that complications can happen. These complications can include injury to the bladder, puncture of a major vessel possibly because a second trocar was not being visualized during placement, or unrecognized injury to bowel because placement of a Verres needle was not properly tested to check for stool.

There are certain points that might be considered important while performing and then transcribing the medico-legal document of operative laparoscopy. The following operations will begin with the basic diagnostic laparoscopy transcription then will become more specific for each individual operative procedure (in order to decrease redundance).

In all laparoscopic operations, stick to the basics and do not forget to transcribe them...

Whenever laparoscopy is employed, videoendoscopy is utilized (if possible). This is certainly not required or recommended, but advantages are 1) allows greater involvement by the operating room team, 2) allows assistants to really "help" or "do more", 3) teaching potential improved, 4) educational tapes can be produced, 5) patient enlightenment, 6) increases referrals for surgery, and 7) makes possible better medico-legal documentation. Some institutions, however, are not equipped with videolaparoscopy therefore for the purpose of this book transcription will be directed to "direct" or "video" visualization. Once familiar with video equipment, the operator can usually perform the entire surgery by watching the video screen without ever having to bend or look through the scope. However, a beam splitter can be advantageous over a direct coupler for video, since the beam splitter allows the operator to view directly in the pelvis but still obtain a good view on the monitor. This is very helpful when first beginning advanced laparoscopic surgeries.

There are many other important points to remember in performing laparoscopic operations which include constant irrigation fluid and/or smoke, being familiar with the equipment, and achieving adequate experience to be able to accomplish good results without too many complications. It is imperative, however, during and after this "learning curve" that these possible complications be recognized if at all possible. It is also possible to reduce the number of complications if certain procedures are routine. This is another purpose of this book – to drill some of these "routine" procedures into a "form" transcription that one can read, perform, and transcribe over and over until these are automatic.

Important points

- If a D&C is performed in conjunction with a laparoscopy – remember to be cautious for false passage ways and post menopausal or postpartum (boggy) uteri that perforate easily.
- Always empty the bladder with catheter prior to placing the Verres needle to decrease chances of inadvertent entry into the urinary bladder.
- Describe the type of trocars used such as disposable, sleeve retractable (Surgiport), long etc...
- Describe the method or methods to test the placement of the initial needle puncture. Methods include:

  a) "Hanging drop method" – place one drop on hub of Verres needle and if it disappears down the needle, it indicates negative intraabdominal cavity pressure.

  b) "Syringe Method" – should indicate no resistance upon pushing the plunger with a few ml of sterile water into the abdomen.

  c) "Bubble Method" – upon pulling the plunger of the sterile water filled syringe back, bubbles should be noted rather than urine, feces, or blood!

  d) "Gas Pressure Gauge Method" – the CO_2 insufflator should not be in the red area or at a more than normal increased pressure (as would be noted if bowel, subcutaneous tissue, or other structures were against the bevel of the needle).

  e) It is not necessary to use towel clips to lift the abdomen for insertion of any trocar.

f) Insert the trocar at the proper angle! Vessels lie deep!

g) Watch *carefully* through the eyepiece or on the video screen when inserting the laparoscope through the sleeve. Laparoscopes can puncture cecums, omentums, and other structures that a sleeve may be directly against.

h) Identify any injuries and correct these at the time of surgery. If there are no injuries and hemostasis is excellent, transcribe these observations.

i) Do not risk causing an ectopic pregnancy or endometriosis. If chromotubation is planned, recommend surgery between the sixth and tenth day of the patient's cycle (if at all possible). This will avoid pushing endometrium or egg backwards through the tubes.

- Beware of Single Puncture Laparoscopic Procedures – under normal operative conditions, a 5 mm instrument protruding 10 mm or more beyond the distal end of the laparoscope will obstruct 14.6% of the operator's visual field.

- Physicians performing laparoscopic procedures must be able to perform the same procedure using open surgery methods in case of emergency.

- Carefully screen patients for laparoscopic surgery. Patients who are significantly overweight or have had previous abdominal incisions are not good candidates for your initial procedures.

- Avoid inadequate insufflation of the patient's abdomen. This will result in collapse of the abdominal wall, increasing the risk of trocar injuries to the abdominal cavity.

- Avoid excessive insufflation of the patient's abdomen (above 20 ml of mercury). This can result in carbon dioxide embolus.

- Do not blindly insert the trocar. Trocars blindly inserted above the patient's midline can result in injury to the iliac or epigastric vessels. Instead use the open technique to make the incision and insert the trocar with direct vision or visualize the insertion via video if available.

- Perform your first 10–20 procedures under the guidance and supervision of a physician who has already mastered laparoscopic techniques. (The majority of all laparoscopic accidents occur during a physician's first 10 procedures.)

- In procedures that last longer than 30 minutes, use

prophylaxis (hose, compression stockings) to prevent pulmonary embolism. In high-risk cases, administer subcutaneous heparin during the procedure.

• Inform patients that laparoscopy, compared to open surgery, may pose additional risks, and explain those risks in appropriate detail. Also tell patients that switching to the open procedure is appropriate if technical problems occur during laparoscopy.

• Key to success of operative laparoscopy is proper placement of second, third, and sometimes fourth ancillary puncture sites which should be anterior and to either side of the tissue of interest, avoiding obstruction of the surgeon's vision or at an angle of poor visibility.

ADHESIOLYSIS (LAPAROSCOPIC LYSIS OF ADHESIONS)

Technique

Aquadissection was performed using the tip of the _____ (Nezhat irrigator, aquadissector) placed against the adhesive interface. The pressurized fluid created a cleavage plane that was able to be extended with further increased fluid pressure and blunt dissection. (Describe whether bowel-adnexa, tube-ovary, adnexa, pelvic sidewall, etc... are being elevated and separated from each other.)

Sharp dissection using _____ (5 or 3 mm) hooked scissors was performed to lyse adhesions that were present between the tube and ovary. Vasopressin (20 U in 50 ml of Ringer's lactate solution) was used to promote hemostasis.

Electro dissection was performed using a (an) _____ (Elmore's, needle electrode, or other standard electrosurgical unit) and 3 mm laparoscopic scalpel with a cutting current of _____ (50-80 W) to divide dense adhesions. Bipolar desiccation at _____ (25 W) was used to control arteriolar bleeding.

CO_2 laser vaporization was also used interchangeable with the electrosurgical equipment. Aquadissection was utilized as a "backstop" by injecting fluid behind the adhesions during the lyses procedure. _____ (14 W) of power was delivered to the tissue using a _____ (5 mm) operating channel in a _____ (40 W) superpulse mode with a _____ (1 mm) spot size.

At the end of the procedure, hemostasis was confirmed with "underwater" examination by filling the pelvis with Ringer's lactate solution and all structures were examined for bleeding. (If there is any bleeding – describe and coagulate with microbipolar forceps.) Prior to closure of the peritoneum, 2000 ml of Ringer's lactate solution was left in the pelvis to separate the structures during the initial stages of reperitonealization.

Author's notes

Transcribe the usual laparoscopic procedure for placement of laparoscopic instrumentation (this can be found in the transcription sample of diagnostic laparoscopy). Usually if adhesions are expected to be severe a vertical intraumbilical incision is made so as to accommodate a 10 mm laparoscope that can be attached to beamsplitter and video. Two additional 5 mm punctures are carried out along the pubic hairline after each has been visualized during placement.

If suturing is required to evert tubal ostia, excise omentum, etc. a modified half-hitch knot is tied loosely allowing the knot to slide to the area being sutured, either freely or with help from a 3 mm laparoscopic needle-holder positioned at the lower-quadrant puncture site. The tapered 1 cm straight needle through a 5 mm short, self-retaining, trapless trocar sleeve is already inside the peritoneal cavity. #0 catgut or 4-0 polydioxanone have been used for this method. Endoloops are preferred by some if free ties can be used.

ADNEXAL TORSION

Technique

Conservative Management Technique A&B; Two additional 5 mm second puncture trocars were inserted in the suprapubic line under (direct or video) _____ visualization. The affected adnexa was untwisted gently with atraumatic laparoscopic forceps to avoid any additional adnexal damage.

Management Technique C; Gangrenous _____ (right, left or both) adnexa was noted and there was no recovery after untwisting and observation for ten minutes.

Author's notes

Transcribe the usual laparoscopic procedure for placement of laparoscopic instrumentation (see diagnostic laparoscopy).

Group A adnexa demonstrates no ischemia or mild lesions with immediate and complete recovery. Group B are tubes and/

or ovaries that demonstrate dark red or black ischemia but with partial recovery approximately ten minutes after the pedicles were untwisted. Whichever findings are noted are described but Group B lesions should undergo a second look laparoscopy six to eight weeks after the initial procedure to assess recovery.)

The majority of torsion cases were caused by ovarian and/or para ovarian cysts. Some of the etiologies can be abnormal length of the uteroovarian ligaments. The cyst can be managed according to descriptions in this book. Laparoscopic ovariopexies can be performed, using Fallopian Rings to shorten the uteroovarian ligament if it is too long, such as described in similar manner to shortening of the round ligaments for laparoscopic uterine suspension.)

Adnexa are usually removed laparoscopically or by laparotomy in scenarios such as seen in group C ... describe and transcribe treatment.

APPENDECTOMY

Technique

The appendix was lifted into view of the video camera using the laparoscopic grasper. The mesoappendiceal vessels were skeletonized by blunt dissection and occluded with 9 mm titanium clips using the ENDO-Clip applier as was necessary. Once the appendix was free, the appendix was measured in thickness and then using the _____ (gray, white) indicator, the appropriately measured multi-fire ENDO GIA 30 was placed across the appendiceal base and fired. The appendix was then released by the grasper, and the multi-fire ENDO GIA 30 was removed and a 5 mm grasper was placed through the 12 mm trocar using a reducer plate to prevent the escape of CO_2. The appendix was then withdrawn totally intact through the 12 mm trocar without difficulty.

The appendiceal stump was inspected closely to insure hemostasis and was irrigated with an antibiotic solution consisting of _____ (2 gms Mandol in 1000 cc normal saline).

Author's notes

Transcribe the usual procedure for a diagnostic laparoscopy except use a 12 mm Surgiport trocar rather than the customary 5 mm suprapubic port, along with right and/or left lower quadrant 5 mm trocars, approximately 10 cm from the midline at a level midway between the umbilicus and the symphysis pubis.

Cautery and Roeder chromic loops can be used for hemostasis of mesoappendix. The loops may also be used to ligate the appendix prior to transection but these methods are becoming much less necessary with the innovative multi-fire ENDO GIA 30 and ENDO-Clips.

BLADDER SUSPENSION OR BURCH PROCEDURE

Transcribe routine placement of 10 x 12 trocars and 5 mm trocars bilateral to epigastric arteries per routine diagnostic laparoscopy.

Laparoscopic endoshears were used to create a 5 cm incision approximately 2 cm above the symphysis pubis along the anterior peritoneum and into the retropubic space. Bipolar forceps were used at least 2–2.5 cm lateral to the urethra to maintain hemostasis.

Two 1.25 x 1–2 cm of prolene mesh passed through the 10 x 12 trocar and an ethicon endoscopic stapler was used to place a staple into the perivaginal fascia, as the assistant used the index and middle finger in the patient's vagina to lift the urethra–vesical junction to identify the area to place the mesh. Two staples were then placed through the mesh into the center of Cooper's ligament. The bladder neck was checked to make certain it was at 1 cm from the symphysis pubis. The mesh was trimmed and excess was removed through the trocar.

The same procedure was performed on the opposite side. The retropubic space was irrigated liberally with RL solution, bleeding points identified, and controlled with bipolar forceps.

Peritoneum was reapproximated with an endopath endoscopic articulating stapler. Trocars were removed as the abdomen and pelvis were inspected. These areas were found to be free of any injury, bleeding, or complication. The punctures were reapproximated with fine 3-0 _____ suture.

CYSTECTOMY

Technique

The cystic capsule was incised with _____ (scissors, laser, or unipolar electrode). A plane was found between the ovarian capsule and the cyst wall. Using the two lower abdominal 5 mm ports, graspers were used to peel back the capsule and the cyst was then teased out of the ovary by traction and counter traction. (This can be accomplished with the cyst intact or after it has been drained.) The cyst was slowly stripped out of the ovary and after it was completely removed, the base was coagulated with _____ (the laser or bipolar forcep). The cyst was then removed by twisting it to allow compression of the tissue and then withdrawn through the _____ (10, 11, or 12 mm) sleeve. Copious irrigation was then utilized throughout the ovary and pelvis. Hemostasis was excellent and there was no injury to any pelvic structures. (A larger cyst or dermoid may be removed with a sac or through a colpotomy.) Instrumentation was removed, incisions reapproximated with _____ (3-0 delayed or 4-0 delayed absorbable) suture and Neosporin with _____ bandaids applied.

Author's notes

Document in transcription the result of the serum Ca-125, the absence of internal or external papillations on pre-op ultrasound, and make certain that proper work-up/documentation was present preoperatively to indicate laparoscopic removal of cyst.

Transcribe routine method of laparoscopic placement of trocars, CO_2, and pelvic findings.

DIAGNOSTIC LAPAROSCOPY

Technique

The patient was prepped with _____ solution and draped in the lithotomy position with special attention to the area of the umbilicus and cervix. Weighted speculum was placed into the vagina so as to expose the cervix. A _____ tenaculum was placed into the cervix to enable the uterus to be manipulated. The weighted speculum was removed and the bladder was emptied with a _____ catheter. Gloves were then changed prior to abdominal incision.

A small subumbilical incision was performed and _____ (Surgiport) Verres needle was placed into the incision and checked by the syringe, the hanging drop, the bubble, and the gas pressure register methods. All methods indicated proper placement of the needle.

Pneumoperitoneum of approximately three liters of CO_2 was established then _____ trocar was properly inserted into the abdomen. The sound of escaping gas confirmed proper location in the abdomen as the trocar was removed from the sleeve.

Fiberoptics (and videocamera if available) were connected to the laparoscope and this was inserted through the sleeve under _____ (direct or video) laparoscopic visualization. Trendelenburg position was increased and approximately one to one and a half liters more of CO_2 gas was allowed into the abdomen to displace the viscera so as to easily visualize the pelvic organs. (Describe the findings.)

The procedure was discontinued and the abdomen was inspected. Hemostasis was excellent. There was no apparent injury to any bladder, bowel, vessels, or other visceral structures. The CO_2 was released from the abdominal cavity. All instrumentation was removed from the abdomen. The subumbilical incision was reapproximated with a figure-of-eight suture utilizing 3-0 _____ suture. Neosporin and bandaid were applied to the incision. All instrumentation was removed from the vagina and the patient went to the Recovery Room in excellent condition.

ECTOPIC PREGNANCY – AMPULLARY SUCTION AND IRRIGATION

Author's notes

Transcribe routine method of laparoscopic placement of trocars, CO_2, and pelvic findings.

Technique

After finding the ectopic pregnancy near the ampulla, the tube was stabilized with an atraumatic grasper through the 5 mm port. Atraumatic grasping forceps were pushed into the tube and prongs were opened to grasp the protruding ectopic. A small Nezhat irrigating and smoke evacuating system was utilized to obtain residual trophoblastic tissue from the end of the tube. Hemostasis was _____ excellent. (Although bleeding rarely occurs, it may be controlled be microbipolar forceps coagulation.) Approximately _____ (500–1000 ml) of lactated Ringer's solution was placed in the pelvis for floatation then CO_2 released from the abdomen after making certain of hemostasis and absence of injury. Instrumentation was removed, incisions reapproximated with _____ , and _____ (dressings, Neosporin, bandaids) applied.

ECTOPIC PREGNANCY – CHEMOTHERAPY OF UNRUPTURED TUBAL PREGNANCY

Author's notes

Transcribe routine method of laparoscopic placement of trocar and/or trocars and CO_2. Transcribe the pelvic findings and describe which tube the ectopic pregnancy was found. Mention that the abnormal pregnancy is 4 cm or less and also make note of the HCG level. It is also suggested to have sonographic evidence especially if video equipment is not available.

Technique

A dilute solution of _____ (vasopressin 20 units in 6 cc NS or Pitressin 0.5–1.0 IV) was injected gently into the mesosalpinx through a _____ (21-gauge) injection needle. _____ (10 cc) of methotrexate solution was injected gently at _____ (five or six) points between the tubal wall and the conceptus. (The dose of methotrexate given at first is 25 mg and amounts then decreased gradually thereafter to the final dose of 5 mg. A 50 mg dose vial is used so that 4 cc of NS is mixed with 1 cc of the 50 mg dose vial. This is usually injected first. Then 4 more cc of normal saline are mixed with the remaining 1 cc of 50 mg dose vial for final injections. Doses of methotrexate can range from as small as 5-25 mg.)

After hemostasis was judged to be excellent the procedure was discontinued. All instrumentation was removed from the abdomen after as much of the CO_2 was removed as possible. (3-0 chromic) suture on an _____ (M-04) needle was used to close the subumbilical and lower abdominal incisions. Vaginal instrumentation was then removed.

ECTOPIC PREGNANCY – SALPINGECTOMY (SEGMENTAL RESECTION)

Author's note

Usually if the fallopian tube is severely damaged or contains an ectopic pregnancy larger than 3 cm, removing the tube or portion of the tube may be easier, safer, and may provide better assurance of complete evacuation of the problem than salpingotomy. Future microsurgical anastomosis can restore potency if only segmental resection is done. Document the reasoning of performing salpingectomy, transcribe routine laparoscopic placement of CO_2 and trocars and then the following.

Technique

The _____ (right or left) tube was free of bowel and other structures. (If the tube is adherent to the bowel or other structures, laparotomy is mandatory in most cases as the mesosalpinx has to be accessible.) With the 10 mm operating laparoscope and two lower operating trocar sheaths in place, the proximal portion of the tube was grasped with laparoscopic flat duck billed bipolar forceps and there cauterized for approximately ten seconds. The fallopian tube was then grasped again along the distal end of the affected area of the tube and again cauterized for approximately ten seconds.

The laparoscopic scissors were placed through the operating sheath in place of the bipolar forceps and the cauterized portions of the tube were transected. The _____ (tube or tubal segment) was grasped with laparoscopic forceps through the 5 mm sheath and the bipolar forceps and scissors were used to alternately cauterize and cut the mesosalpinx beneath the affected tube.

The _____ (affected segment or tube) was then seized by one end with a forcep placed through the laparoscope's operating channel. It was then carefully removed with the laparoscope through the sheath. (The tube or tubal segment may need to be divided into fragments if it is so large as to prevent passage of the tube through the 10 mm sheath.)

There was no injury to the pelvis, hemostasis was excellent, and CO_2 was released from the abdominal cavity as all instrumentation was removed from the abdomen. The incisions were reapproximated with _____ (3-0 delayed absorbable) suture.

_____ (Neosporin) and bandaids were placed over the incisional sites. Vaginal instrumentation was removed and the patient went to the recovery room in good condition. (Overnight observation may sometimes be considered to rule out intraperitoneal bleeding.)

ECTOPIC PREGNANCY – SALPINGOTOMY (FOR REMOVAL OF ECTOPIC PREGNANCY)

Author's notes

Transcribe routine method of laparoscopic placement of trocars, CO_2, and pelvic findings.

Technique

After placement of additional lower abdominal trocars in the midline and near the hairline lateral to the inferior epigastric artery, the tube was stabilized with an atraumatic grasper. The mesosalpinx was injected with a vasopressin (20 units/100 ml) solution. This was accomplished by placing a long spinal needle directly through the skin of the abdomen and into the mesosalpinx taking care to avoid blood vessels. Approximately _____ (10 ml) was injected. The fallopian tube was then incised directly over the ectopic bulge along the antimesenteric border. The incision was performed with a _____ (unipolar electrode needle or knife, or with a laser). After a short time, the conceptus began to extrude through the opening of the tube. The remainder was _____ (irrigated out using a Nezhat hydrosurgical irrigator or teasing it out with small grasping forceps) through the 5 mm port. The tissue was then removed through the _____ (10/12 mm) midline port using a _____ (spoon forcep or endopouch).

The tube and pelvis was then thoroughly irrigated with copious amounts of sterile _____ (fluid) until clear. The salpingotomy incision was left open. Hemostasis was _____ (excellent, etc...). (If there is any bleeding along the tube, one suture of PDS, 4-0 Vicryl, or a small bipolar coagulator may be used to bring about hemostasis.) The laparoscopy was completed, no injury to any structures were found, CO_2 was released, instrumentation removed under _____ (direct or video) laparoscopic vision, and the incisions were reapproximated and dressed appropriately.

Serial quantitative beta-HCG level was drawn in the recovery room and the patient was given instructions to return weekly for repeat levels until persistent trophoblastic disease or pregnancy is ruled out.

ENDOMETRIOSIS

Overview

Endometriosis may be treated by many methods including excision, unipolar or bipolar electro-coagulation, laser vaporization, hormonal therapy, thermocoagulation, and for larger lesions such as endometrioma – either removal or opening and draining of the lesions with minimal intracavitary manipulation except washing. Thermocoagulation or laser therapy will be used here only because of the author's preference, need for brievity, and the belief that these modalities are probably safer than electrocautery because of the area of destruction around the coagulation point being smaller than unipolar or bipolar electrocoagulation. When laser is mentioned, CO_2 or Nd:YAG (with sapphire tip) are preferred because of their depths of penetration yet depth of lateral damage being held at a minimum of around 400–800 microns. A sample finding for this particular transcription will be included so as to demonstrate various examples of endometriosis treatment.

Technique

An endometrioma of the right ovary was noted measuring 3 cm in size. There were other nonspecific lesions that appeared to be endometriosis of the cul-de-sac and left ovary. The right ovary also appeared to be adhered to the uterosacral ligament and right pelvic side wall.

Keeping the foot "very light" on the _____ (laser, coagulator) pedal, the right ovary was systematically lysed away from areas of the rectum and ureter being very careful to avoid these structures. The _____ (Nezhat) suction irrigation probe was used to bluntly lyse these adhesions and thus lift up the ovary. An initial incision was carried out into the right ovary using the _____ (laser) on _____ (superpulse 3, spot size 0.5, fast mode). The relaxing incision was then carried out in a circular fashion _____ (2-4 mm) around the initial incision. Using two sets of grasping forceps through the 5 mm ports, the lesion was then stripped away from the healthy ovarian tissue. This was then brought through the _____ (10 mm/12 mm) port. Hemostasis was excellent. Irrigation was placed into the cavity using Ringer's lactate solution.

The 3 mm knife electrode was used to incise and drain areas of the left ovary with superficial endometriosis and deeper cysts suspicious for endometrioma. A cyst cavity was discovered in one area and this was irrigated with Ringer's lactate solution and then excised in the same manner as was performed on the _____ (right, opposite) ovary using 3 mm and 5 mm grasping forceps. The ovary fell back together naturally after removal of the cyst wall. The remainder of very small lesions, less than 1 cm, were fulgurated with a 3 mm _____ (point, hook) electrode.

Excision of several of the larger implants in the cul-de-sac were excised using the _____ (CO_2) laser using a spot size of _____ and power density of _____ (as high as possible) to vaporize the margins of the lesion preserving the lesion itself. These were removed through the _____ (5 mm, 10 mm, or 12 mm) port. The remainder of the lesions less than 2 mm were vaporized with the laser or coagulated with the _____ (point thermo-coagulator or bipolar coagulator).

After the entire pelvis was inspected and found to have no other pathology indicative of endometriosis, hemostasis and absence of inadvertent injury was assured, and pneumo-peritoneum was released from the abdomen. Abdominal instrumentation was removed under _____ (direct or video) visualization. Incisions were reapproximated using _____ (3-0 or 4-0 delayed absorbable) suture. _____ (Neosporin) and _____ (bandaids) were placed over the incisions. Vaginal instrumentation was removed. The patient went to the recovery room in excellent condition.

Author's notes

Transcribe the usual procedure for a diagnostic laparoscopy with the addition of 12 mm and bilateral lower 5 mm port placements if needed.

HYSTERECTOMY (LAPAROSCOPIC ASSISTED VAGINAL HYSTERECTOMY)

Technique

Patient was prepped and draped with Betadine in the lithotomy position. The weighted speculum was placed into the vagina and a single tooth tenaculum was utilized on the anterior lip of the cervix. The tenaculum was placed into the intrauterine cavity and the uterus was stabilized. Ureteral catheters were bilaterally placed cystoscopically *(this is done if ureters are not dissected into view laparoscopically)*. The single tooth tenaculum was removed and all retractors removed. A catheter was placed with Foley bag and attention was placed on the abdomen. Gloves were changed. A small subumbilical incision was carried out and Surgiport Verres needle was placed in the routine manner. Placement was checked by the hanging drop method, the syringe method, gas pressure register method, and the bubble method. Pneumoperitoneum of approximately 3 liters of CO_2 was established and the laparoscopic _____ (10,11, or 10/12 mm) trocar was placed in the routine manner withdrawing the trocar listening for sound of escaping gas for confirmation of proper location. Video fiberoptics were connected and the videoscope was gently inserted under direct video laparoscopic visualization. Trendelenburg position was increased and approximately 1.5 liters more of gas was allowed into the abdomen to better displace the viscera so as to easily visualize the pelvic organs. *(Describe gross pathology.)* The 5 mm trocar incisors were made in the lower abdomen and 5 mm laparoscopic trocars were placed visualizing the placement via video camera during the entire procedure. A small midline incision was carried out approximately 5 to 10 cm below the umbilicus and a 12 mm trocar was placed through this incision under direct video laparoscopic visualization. There appeared to be no complications during placement of extra trocars. A 5 mm laparoscopic grasper was utilized to lift the right ovary and fallopian tube toward the midline. Endogage was secured to determine whether a 3.5 or 3 V staple size should be used. Through the 12 mm trocar sleeve, a GIA-30 was placed and the infundibulopelvic ligament was clamped and cut in one motion using GIA-30. The staple line was examined for clip placement and hemostasis. The round, broad, and utero-ovarian ligaments were also clamped with the GIA-30 and manipulated so that the grasper held the ovary and fallopian tube in place in order to make placement easy. Following the removal of the right ovary and tube, a 5 mm grasper was placed through an adaptor on the 12 mm trocar following removal of the GIA-30 instrumentation. The ovary and tube were pulled up through the _____ (12, 18 mm) sleeve. The same procedure was performed on the left side as was on the right in that the 5 mm laparoscopic grasper was used to manipulate the left ovary and tube in order to place another GIA-30 through the 12 mm sleeve so as to clamp and cut the left infundibulopelvic ligament. The ovary and tube were then removed through the _____ (12, 18 mm) sleeve. The staple line was inspected and found to be hemostatic. There appeared to be no injury to any abdominal viscera. The round, broad, and utero-ovarian ligaments were then bilaterally clamped and cut using the GIA-30 through the 12 mm sleeve and then the bladder flap was developed using the distal clips at the bottom of the broad ligaments as left and right markers. The flap was created using (laparoscopic scissors or contact laser technique with the 0.6 mm-scalpel tip or chisel tip at a power setting of 15 watts), thus exposing the anterior cul-de-sac. The ureteral catheters were continually moved and palpated so as to identify the ureters. The uterosacral ligaments were then transected using _____ (the Endo-GIA stapler or Nd: YAG laser with chisel tip). With moist sponge on a sponge stick and posterior to the cervix, a colpotomy was performed with _____ (the contact laser scalpel or scissors) by incising between the uterosacral ligaments. Pneumoperitoneum was then lost and attention was then directed to the vaginal portion of the procedure. After appropriate vaginal exposure, anterior colpotomy was performed and uterus removed. Vaginal cuff was reapproximated with _____ (0-delayed absorbable) suture in hemostatic fashion. Pneumoperitoneum was reestablished, and vaginal cuff and staple lines were inspected for tissue approximation and hemostasis. All instrumentation was then removed and incisions reapproximated with _____ (3-0 chromic) suture. Neosporin and bandaids were applied over incisions.

MYOMECTOMY

Two sample transcriptions are presented here as there are different circumstances of myoma.

Technique I

The myoma was grasped with a _____ ("double-toothed biopsy forceps" or, if the myoma is too large for forceps to hold, with a "claw forceps"), through the 5 mm port. The stalk was then grasped with a crocodile forceps and carefully coagulated from all sides for approximately 30 seconds until hemostasis was thought to be assured. The myoma was then excised with laparoscopic hook scissors. Oozing was controlled with the _____ (point coagulator or laser). The myoma was then removed directly with the claw forceps through the 12 mm trocar sleeve. Thorough irrigation was then performed throughout the pelvis.

Author's note

If necessary morcellation and extraction or colpotomy can be performed for large myomata.

Technique II

After estimating the myoma's size and extent, 5 U of vasopressin in 100 ml of normal saline was injected into the base and capsule. Another 5-10 ml of the vasopressin was then carefully injected into the corner of each side of the uterus (to constrict the ascending branch of the uterine artery). Once the myoma was noted to be white due to ischemia, enucleation of the myoma was started.

The serosal capsule was endocoagulated with the point coagulator in a 4 mm wide band. The capsule was then incised with the laparoscopic _____ (hook, micro) scissors (or laser beam) to establish a cleavage plane.

The capsule was then systematically stripped off the myoma using the enucleator (heated to 120 °C). The myoma was stabilized with a (myoma cork screw or large claw forceps). Once the base was reached, care was taken not to lacerate the feeding vessels.

The myoma was then removed by placing _____ (an endoloop, Roeder loop, or endoligature) around the base through the 5 mm port and securely ligating the feeding vessels so as to prevent retraction. The pedicle was then cut with hook scissors above the point of ligation. The myoma was detached by _____ (twisting or coagulating) the pedicle. The crater was then thoroughly irrigated with normal saline and inspected for hemostasis. The point coagulator was used as necessary. Interceed was then placed over the area. (If the crater was large) – an endosuture with a 3 mm needle holder was loaded into a suture applicator. The applicator was then fed through the lower abdominal 5 mm trocar. A 5 mm needle holder was then placed through the contralateral 5 mm port and used to pick up the needle, bring out to tie a slip knot, then pushed back into the pelvis with a push rod attached to the ligature to reapproximate the serosal capsule walls. Irrigation was again performed after suturing was completed using _____ (#) interrupted sutures of (4-0 to 6-0 PDS, etc).

The myoma was then _____ (morcellated or extracted through a posterior colpotomy or 12 mm port).

After assessing that hemostasis was excellent, and that no injury had occurred to other structures – pneumoperitoneum was released and instrumentation removed under _____ (direct or video) visualization. Reapproximation of the incisions with _____ suture, placement of bandaids, and removal of vaginal instrumentation completed the operation.

Author's notes

Embedded myoma cannot initially be grasped. This requires dissection of the capsule then corkscrew placement for further dissection.

If the base or pedicle is not considered very large and hemostasis is not much of concern, one may transcribe the following for removal; 'the myoma was detached by _____ (twisting or coagulating) the pedicle.'

If coagulation was performed, simply transcribe: 'hook scissors were then used to cut the pedicle.'

It is sometime recommended to place a Robinson drain through a lower abdominal 5 mm port and into the cul-de-sac for approximately 24 h following removal of the myoma or myomae.

NEOSALPINGOTOMY (VIDEOLASER LAPAROSCOPIC NEOSALPINGOTOMY)

Technique

The patient was prepped with solution and draped in the lithotomy position with special attention to the area of the umbilicus and cervix. Weighted speculum was placed into the vagina so as to expose the cervix. A Hume tenaculum with cannula was placed into the cervix to enable the uterus to be manipulated and chromotubation to be performed. The weighted speculum was removed and the bladder was emptied with a _____ catheter. Adapter tubing with indigo carmine in a 60 cc syringe was attached to the cannula for injection of blue dye. Gloves were then changed prior to abdominal incision.

A small subumbilical incision was performed and _____ (Verres) needle was placed into the incision and checked by the syringe, the hanging drop, the bubble, and the gas pressure register methods. All methods indicated proper placement of the needle.

Pneumoperitoneum of approximately 3 liters of CO_2 was established then _____ trocar was properly inserted into the abdomen. The sound of escaping gas confirmed proper location in the abdomen as the trocar was removed from the sleeve.

Fiberoptics (and videocamera if available) were connected to the laparoscope and this was inserted through the sleeve under _____ (direct or video) laparoscopic visualization. Trendelenburg position was increased and approximately 1–1.5 liters more of CO_2 gas was allowed into the abdomen to displace the viscera so as to easily visualize the pelvic organs. (Describe the findings.) Chromotubation was performed to inspect tubal blockage.

After confirmation of the _____ (right, left, or bilateral) hydrosalpinx was made, a second puncture was carried out for the placement of the Nezhat smoke – evacuator and aquadissector. A third puncture was then carried out along the opposite lower abdominal quadrant for placement of an accessory forcep to be used for traction and tubal manipulation. Both second and third punctures of trocars and sleeves were performed under _____ (direct or video) visualization to insure against an unrecognized visceral injury.

The _____ (CO_2, Argon, KTP) laser was set on _____ (usually high wattage of about 24–30 watts with use of a superpulse mode). The laser was used initially over the thinnest portion of the distal tube making an incision with the use of two grasping forceps for traction and counter traction. The tube immediately collapsed as the blue dye inside the tube flowed out. Radial cuts were then made along the tube using a backstop probe being careful throughout the operation to avoid the thicker portion of the tube and stay clear of the mesenteric border where larger vessels were located.

After the radial incisions had been made, the tubal edges were everted outwards by setting the laser on 2–3 W in a defocused mode and firing the laser beam several cm from the lateral peritoneal edge of the distal tube. The results were like outward petals of a flower.

Copious irrigation with heparinized (5000 units per liter) Ringer's lactate was performed through the Nezhat irrigator over the entire flowered back fallopian tube. Hemostasis was excellent. Chromotubation was then done and tuboscopy was performed with saline for tubal dilatation to evaluate the status of the endothelium of the ampullary portion of the tube. The amount of destruction was considered _____ (minimal, moderate, or severe). The patient's prognosis was considered _____ for pregnancy after the surgery.

The procedure was discontinued and the abdomen was inspected. Hemostasis was excellent. There was no apparent injury to any bladder, bowel, vessels, or other visceral structures. The CO_2 was released from the abdominal cavity. All instrumentation was removed from the abdomen. The subumbilical incision was reapproximated with a figure-of-eight suture utilizing 3-0 _____ suture. Neosporin and bandaid were applied to the incision. All instrumentation was removed from the vagina and the patient went to the Recovery Room in excellent condition.

Author's notes

CO_2 laser can be used with this technique but it is easier to perform with the use of an argon or KTP laser – it is suggested that the type of laser be mentioned in the operative report.

OOPHORECTOMY (LAPAROSCOPIC SALPINGO-OOPHORECTOMY – RIGHT, LEFT OR BILATERAL)

Technique

The decision to possibly remove the _____ (right ovary and tube) had been made previously with the patient prior to the procedure. A 5 mm trocar was placed in the lower right abdominal quadrant and was visualized during the videolaparoscopy. Another incision was made in the middle lower abdomen between the symphysis pubis and the umbilicus in order to place the 12 mm laparoscopic trocar. This was also visualized under videolaparoscopy. Through the 5 mm trocar, a laparoscopic grasper was placed and the ovary was lifted into view with the grasper. Through the 12 mm sleeve a GIA 30 multi-fire unit was placed at the base of the ovary and fallopian tube along the utero-ovarian and infundibulopelvic ligament. The instrument was fired and released. Another GIA 30 multi-fire unit was then placed through the 12 mm sleeve and again placed at the base of the ligaments and fired. This allowed the fallopian tube and the ovary to be dislodged from their ligaments.

A 5 mm adaptor to insure no escape of CO_2 was placed over the 12 mm trocar and a 5 mm laparoscopic grasper was placed through this and the ovary was grasped and pulled to the 12 mm trocar sleeve. The fallopian tube was able to be brought up into the 12 mm sleeve, but the ovary was unable to be pulled into the sleeve. Therefore, the sleeve was pulled up through the incision and once the sleeve was removed from the incision, the fallopian tube was in view of the skin. Using forceps, the fallopian tube and ovary were worked through the skin until the entire ovary and fallopian tube had been removed from the incision (see Author's note).

It was at this point that the procedure was discontinued and the abdomen was inspected while pulling the trocars out. Hemostasis was excellent and there was no apparent injury to any bladder, bowel, vessels, or visceral structures. The CO_2 was released from the abdominal cavity. All instrumentation was removed from the abdomen. The subumbilical incision was reapproximated with a figure-of-eight suture utilizing _____ (3-0 chromic) suture. The other two incisions were also reapproximated with _____ (3-0 chromic) suture. Neosporin and bandaids were applied over each incision. All instrumentation was removed from the vagina and the patient went to the Recovery Room in excellent condition.

Author's notes

Transcribe routine entry and operative report for diagnostic laparoscopy prior to other trocar placements.

A 5 mm trocar is placed in the lower right abdominal quadrant and *visualized during videolaparoscopy* in order to insure proper placement and to insure there is no injury to abdominal viscera.

An alternate method to remove the ovary (see second paragraph) is to transcribe: 'The ovary was cut with laparoscopic scissors by holding the ovary up against the barrel of the 12 mm sleeve until the ovary had been elongated in order to slide up through the 12 mm sleeve.' A morcellator may also be used if necessary. An *endocatch* bag is often helpful to remove adnexa that are difficult to pull up through the 12 mm sleeve.

It is sometimes necessary to place the 5 mm trocar in the lower abdominal quadrant opposite to the adnexa to be removed, according to the operator's preference.

TUBO-OVARIAN ABSCESS (TOA)

Overview

After presumptive diagnosis of TOA, arrange hospitalization for laparoscopy. The average rate of misdiagnosis of PID, as confirmed by laparoscopy, has been estimated as high as 35%. Even a seemingly obvious TOA may prove to be an endometrioma, hemorrhagic corpus luteum cyst, or abscess surrounding a ruptured appendix.

Reich described the role of laparoscopy in treating TOA and pelvic abscess in an Update on Surgery in Contemporary OB/ GYN in 1989. He recommended that antibiotics be started usually 2–24 hours prior to laparoscopy. He recommended cefoxitin 2 g with oral doxycycline on postoperative day 1. Droegemueller recommends a regimen of clindamycin and gentamycin if abscess is suspected.

Reich offers that the advantages of laparoscopy over laparotomy includes less blood loss using the Aquapurator, *less* superficial and deep wound infection, dehiscence, bowel injury, bowel obstruction, persistent undrained pus collections, thrombophlebitis, pulmonary embolism, septic shock, and subdiaphragmatic abscess.

Author's notes

Transcribe routine technique for diagnostic laparoscopy combined with hysteroscopy during peritoneal insufflation to assess the endometrial cavity and take culture specimens. During the transcription of the laparoscopy and following the hysteroscopy, place a Cohen cannula in the endocervical canal for uterine manipulation and tubal lavage.

Technique

Second and third trocars were placed under _____ (direct or video) visualization just below the pubic hairline adjacent to the inferior epigastric vessels. A _____ (blunt probe or grasping forceps) were inserted through the right-sided trocar sleeve to be used for traction and retraction. A _____ (Nezhat irrigation/ suction probe or Aquapurator) was inserted into the left-sided trocar sleeve. This was utilized to mobilize omentum, small bowel, rectosigmoid, and tubo-ovarian adhesions until entry into the abscess cavity. Purulent fluid was aspirated while returning the patient from 20° to 10° Trendelenburg position. Separate culture of fluid aspirate and inflammatory exudate were obtained and sent to bacteriology.

The _____ (Aquapurator or Nezhat irrigator/suction device) was used to separate bowel and omentum from the uterus and adnexa. It was also used to lyse adhesions. The _____ (Nezhat or Aquapurator's) tip was placed against the adhesive interface between bowel, adnexa, and pelvic sidewall, thus the plane of dissection was extended bluntly using the tip and pressurized fluid stream. Grasping forceps were utilized to place tension on the distorted tissue plane for accurate identification. Necrotic inflammatory tissue and exudate of the abscess cavity was excised with a 5 mm biopsy forceps after dissection was complete. Irrigation of all cavities, holes, and fimbrial ostia were performed with the _____ (Aquapurator or Nezhat irrigator) to remove infected debris and lessen chances of recurrence. This irrigation was performed in a retrograde manner into the fimbrial ostia using grasping forceps to speed away the agglutinating fimbria. The fimbrial mucosa was assessed for its quality for future prognosis which can be described as _____ .

Tubal lavage with indigo carmine through the Cohen cannula was attempted. Patency was _____ (absent or present). (Describe if any inspissated necrotic material was visualized being pushed through the tube.)

Liberal use of lavage was performed using Ringer's lactate until the effluent was clear. Approximately 1 liter of Ringer's lactate was flushed through the _____ (Aquapurator or Nezhat device) on each side of the falciform ligament in the upper abdomen to dilute any purulent material that may have entered these areas during the 20° Trendelenburg positioning. Reverse Trendelenburg position was then used to help suction as much fluid as possible away from the peritoneal cavity.

The laparoscope and irrigation/suction device was then manipulated into the deep cul-de-sac beneath floating bowel and omentum. Irrigation and suction was performed until the effluent was clear. Separation and hemostasis appeared complete.

Approximately 2 liters of fresh irrigant was left in the peritoneal cavity to prevent fibrin adherence between visual structures. There was no apparent injury to any bladder, bowel, vessels, or other visual structures. All instrumentation was removed from the abdomen.

The subumbilical adhesion was reapproximated with a figure-of-eight suture utilizing 3-0 _____ suture. Neosporin and bandaids were applied to the incision. The second and third puncture sites were approximated loosely with a _____ (Javid vascular clamp) to allow drainage of excess irrigant caused by possible intra abdominal pressure. All instrumentation was then removed from the vagina. The patient went to the recovery room in _____ condition.

UTERINE SUSPENSION

Technique

The round ligaments were identified bilaterally. _____ (Two or more) Falope Rings were applied on each round ligament, creating small loops. The round ligaments were noted to be shortened bilaterally, and the uterus was pulled forward. The round ligament appeared to be shortened by about _____ (3 cm).

There appeared to be no transection or bleeding. *(If indeed, there is no bleeding.)*

Author's notes

Transcribe the routine laparoscopic surgery in regards to the evaluation of infertility or pelvic pain and placement of trocars. In a series of 150 patients reported on by Seroor et al, transection and bleeding occurred in 3.33%. *

References

* Seroor GI, Hefnani F: A new approach to the problem of retroverted uterus in infertile patients. Presented at the IXth World Congress of Obstetrics and Gynecology, Tokyo, Oct. 25-31, 1979.

* Seroor GI, Hefnani FI, Handil O, et al: Laparoscopic Ventrosuspension: A new technique. Int. J. Gynaecol. Obstet. 20: 129, 1982.

UTEROSACRAL NERVE ABLATION (LUNA)

Technique

The uterosacral ligaments were placed on stretch by flexing the uterus upwards toward the anterior abdominal wall. The CO_2

laser which was set at _____ (10–20 watts/cm^3) and was fired at the uterosacral ligaments at their insertions into the cervix. Vaporization was limited to the uterosacral ligaments using a back and forth motion of the laser beam. Bleeding was controlled by defocused beams while lasering was kept very superficial.

A superficial vaporization was continued in a "U" shaped fashion across the base of the cervix to connect the two "cut" areas.

Author's notes

Transcribe the usual laparoscopic procedure for placement of laparoscopic instrumentation.

Bleeding is controlled by defocused beams whilst lasering is kept very superficial. This is important to avoid further bleeding and or/or injury to the ureter.

Any treatment of endometriosis, lysis of adhesions, or other surgery should now be completed and transcribed.

Laser procedures

MARSUPIALIZATION OF BARTHOLIN'S GLAND CYST

Technique

After Betadine prep of the _____ (left or right) vulvar area and surrounding vulva and perineum, the colposcopic laser was adjusted to a power density of 900 watts per cm^2 with a 1.5 mm spot size. Using super pulse 2, 0–2 seconds exposure rate, moderate speed; a 1.5 cm oval neostoma was created, extending from the vulvar skin into the cystic cavity, following as closely as possible to the original duct tract. The 1.5 cm defect was created by moving the laser beam rapidly in a circular fashion, thereby vaporizing a cylinder of tissue from the vulva epithelium into the cystic space, resulting in the removal of the obstructed main duct. The cylinder of tissue removed was 1.5 cm in diameter. The beam of application was very precise in that the operating colposcope was used as a microscope by coupling this to the laser. A copious amount of _____ (dark reddish mucus etc.) escaped upon entering the cystic cavity. A routine culture was obtained.

The gland was gently massaged until all free mucus had been expressed. The cystic cavity was irrigated with both sterile normal saline and Betadine, using Q-tips. The lining of the cyst was then inverted and sutured to the vaginal mucosa on both sides with interrupted figure-of-eight sutures of No. 4-0 _____ (absorbable material). Again, the area was thoroughly irrigated with Betadine and no drains or packs were left in place.

The patient has been instructed to refrain from intercourse for approximately two weeks and has been asked to return to the office in approximately six days for a follow-up. Oozing during the procedure was noted interoperatively but was easily controlled by decreasing the power density, beam defocusing, and using pulses. The tongue blade was also used as a back-stop behind the Bartholin's gland to prevent any aberrant reflection of laser beam. The patient was found to be very hemostatic and a very good result was noted. She left the Recovery Room in good condition.

VAPORIZATION OF CERVIX

Technique

The metal bivalve speculum was inserted into the vagina, the cervix was exposed, and local anesthesia was placed in the cervix. The transformational zone and area of pathology were again identified by washing the cervix with a 3% solution of acetic acid. The smoke evacuating system and blood evacuating system was connected to the laser speculum. The laser was placed on a power density of 1800 watts per cm. The power setting was placed on superpulse three with laser beam diameter calculated to be 0.5 mm, exposure rate of 0.2 seconds and with a fast mode of repeat delivery. The entire transformational zone, including the abnormal cytology and flat condyloma, were outlined with the laser beam. The outlined area was divided into four quadrants with short bursts of laser energy. This outline extended approximately 3–4 mm beyond the diseased area in the transformational zone.

Beginning at six o'clock position of the cervix, the laser beam was moved quickly over the tissue to be destroyed in the southwest quadrant. The southeast quadrant was then lasered in the same manner. The northeast and northwest quadrants were then lasered in similar manner. The laser beam was moved in multiple directions, including diagonally, horizontally and vertically. Rapid movement of the beam was utilized. A minimum depth of at least 6 mm was achieved with a 4 mm depth of normal tissue being obtained beyond the lesion and transformational zone. The defect was also lasered centrally incorporating approximately 8–10 mm altitude.

Hemostasis was maintained with the same power density, utilizing a suction device to remove the blood from the operative site, and sometimes increasing the spot size to 2 mm for coagulation. The result was excellent, and the laser char was removed with swabs of 3% acetic acid solution.

The patient has been given routine postoperative instructions and recommendations, including recommendations for mild analgesic, instructions to refrain from intercourse, douching and using tampons for approximately three weeks. She will return for postoperative check-up in three months for repeat cytology and possible repeat colposcopic examination if necessary.

VAPORIZATION OF CONDYLOMA (RECTAL, VULVAR, CERVICAL AND VAGINAL)

Technique

The patient had been previously shaved of hair from the perineum and anal exterior and all external warts were vaporized along the perineum, posterior fourchette and neighboring skin was brushed.

An anal laser speculum was lubricated and placed into the anus. The blades were gently opened and the mucosa was inspected of any visible warts and these were vaporized utilizing low power densities of approximately 350 watts per cm. The speculum was rotated clockwise to cover the entire anus. A wet sponge was placed above to seal the rectum and a vacuum hose was attached to the laser speculum to automatically effect the smoke evacuation.

When anal treatment was completed, a second speculum was placed into the vagina. The cervix was exposed and warty lesions were vaporized along the vagina. Using a long handled spot size laser manipulator of 0.1 mm, the vaginal fornices were exposed and treated. The remaining vaginal walls were examined and treated. Microwarty changes noted on the vagina were also treated on the lateral vaginal walls and brushed by angulating the laser and shooting between the blades of the speculum and the laser beam was reflected as necessary. The hymenal ring and vestibule were also treated.

The cervix was treated under 3% acetic acid solution utilizing the same powered density to vaporize all surface flat condyloma. The procedure was then discontinued, all instrumentation was removed and patient was removed to the Recovery Room in good condition.

VAPORIZATION OF VAIN (VAGINAL INTRAEPITHELIAL NEOPLASIA)

Technique

The laser bivalve speculum and the posterior vaginal cuff was swabbed thoroughly with 5% acetic acid solution (white table vinegar). The cotton tip applicator was moistened with the 5% acetic acid solution and thoroughly swabbed throughout the posterior vaginal area. By withdrawing and rotating the speculum, the vaginal mucosa folded over several times permitting an end-on view of the tissue. The lesions began to appear white and sharply bordered. A power density of 25 watts per cm^2 and then

40 watts per cm² was selected and a spot size of 2 mm was utilized. Utilizing a spinal needle, 2% Xylocaine solution was injected underneath the VAIN lesions and approximately 2 mm of depth was obtained during the laser vaporization to ensure complete vaporization. After outlining each lesion and using the Iris hooks to obtain full vaporizing capacity along the border of normal tissue, the intraepithelial disease was removed using circumferential and cross hatched methods down to the depth in which the lesion was initially achieved when the lesion was outlined.

Hemostasis was achieved by both defocusing the laser beam and also Monsel's solution. The lesions that were involved along the posterior vaginal cuff and hidden by folds, were grasped with the Iris hook and averted so that the lesion could be treated. There was a lesion noted on the _____ (left middle third, for example) of the vagina and vaporization was performed as the tissue folded down over the end of the speculum blades permitting end-on ablation of the lesion. Injection of anesthetic was necessary. There were some small warty lesions over the _____ (left or right third) of the vagina at the introitus and these were treated by passing the laser beam between the blades of the speculum and a small amount of bleeding was controlled by lowering the wattage and placing a small swab of Monsel's solution. After the therapy was completed, the 5% acetic acid solution was used again to inspect the entire vagina and there were no other lesions noted. The procedure was discontinued and the speculum was removed from the vagina. The patient went to the recovery room in good condition and has been given routine discharge instructions and recommendations.

Laparotomy, exploratory

Technique

The patient was prepped and draped _____ (in the routine fashion or as quickly as possible to obtain a sterile field). A (describe incision) incision was carried out along the skin. The subcutaneous fat was incised and fascia then entered. Fascial incision was extended with Mayo scissors. Rectus muscle sheaths were separated in the midline. Peritoneum was picked up with hemostats away from underlying structures. Care was taken while incising the peritoneum with Metzenbaum scissors. The peritoneal incision was then extended with the scissors.

Standing on the patient's right side, the right hand was placed into the upper abdomen. After appropriate washings were obtained (if this step is included), the right kidney, liver, gallbladder, pancreas, stomach, left kidney, and para-aortic lymph nodes were palpated in sequence.

Author's notes

Findings are described and the remainder of the procedure transcribed.

LEEP (conization)

Technique

Bivalve speculum was placed into the vagina and the cervix was swabbed with 4% acetic acid solution. Colposcopy had already been performed. Lugol's solution was placed over the cervix and the limits of the lesion were determined. A solution of 2% Xylocaine with epinephrine, (1 to 100,000) of approximately _____ (9) cc was mixed with 1 cc of sodium bicarbonate. This solution was then used to inject approximately 2 cc deep near the edge of the ATZ circumferentially and approximately 1 mm deep into the cervical stroma around the cervical canal for depth of approximately 1 cm. The antenna plate was placed under the patient. A 2.5 cm electrode was attached to the sterile pencil unit and the current selector was placed on power _____ (#7) at "blend filter-cut". The tip of the loop electrode was moistened. The cervix was also noted to be moist. The loop was slowly moved in a vertical direction from _____ (6 o'clock to 12 o'clock) beyond the edge of the lesion, and with a steady slow motion, the loop was moved beneath the lesion and moved to an exit of _____ (12 o'clock) position without any drag. The excised specimen was removed and sent for pathological evaluation. Bleeding was minimal but it was necessary to use the ball electrode in the setting of coagulation current. Care was taken to avoid coagulating around the endocervical canal. Colposcopy revealed no further persistence of disease. The square electrode was then placed at the _____ (9 o'clock) position and moved to the _____ (3 o'clock) position with approximately 3 to 4 mm away from the canal and a plug of tissue was then removed from the canal. The 4% acetic acid solution was the placed along the crater with a moistened cotton tip applicator to further inspect for residual disease.

There was no further residual signs of disease. The canal appeared to be clear and smooth with a pinkish-orange epithelium. There was no evidence of any white appearing or dense appearing tissue. A ball electrode was used to further coagulate small bleeding points, and then a thick film of Monsel's paste was placed into the crater and held in place for approximately 45 seconds. At this point, hemostasis was judged to be excellent, and all vaginal instrumentation was removed from the vagina.

Patient tolerated the procedure well and went to the Recovery Room in good condition.

Preoperatively, the patient had been given postoperative instructions which included recommendations to refrain from coitus, douching, and tampons for approximately 3 weeks. She was also advised that a brownish-black vaginal discharge would be present for a few days to 2–3 weeks and that if bleeding or spotting persisted longer than 6 days that she should call the office. She will return to the office for a re-pap in approximately 3 months.

Marshall–Marchetti–Krantz procedure

Technique

After the intra-abdominal procedure was performed and completed, semi-frog position under anesthesia and pelvic examination was performed. A #24 Foley catheter with a 5 cc bulb was inserted into the bladder and inflated.

The dissection into the space of Retzius was started after the gloves had been changed and sterile procedure was followed. Any oozing and bleeding that was encountered was controlled by pressure, individual ligature, and careful fulguration. The dissection into the space of Retzius was carried down toward the inferior aspect of the symphysis within 1 cm of the external urethral meatus. After inserting two fingers into the vagina to elevate the anterior vagina and bladder neck so that the sutures could be more easily and accurately placed, the catheter demonstrated the urethra and a balloon indicated the bladder neck and trigonal area. The sutures of #1 _____ (delayed absorbable) material were placed consisting of two sutures on either side. Each suture was taken into the submucosa of the vaginal wall lateral to the urethra, into the fascia adjacent to the wall of the urethra, and then into the fibrocartilage of the symphysis using #4 Mayo round needle. During the placement of the suture the curvature of the needle was followed very accurately to avoid breakage of the needle or laceration of the tissue. The assistant and myself then changed gloves and gown and the sutures were then tied and cut in pairs from below upward.

After adequate suspension a suprapubic Silastic tube (#12 French) was then inserted through the skin and into the bladder under direct vision for abdominal drainage prior to closure of the incision. Two small Penrose drains were placed on either side of the midline in the operative area so as to drain any residual venous bleeding that might occur following closure of the wound. Then, routine closure of the fascia and muscle along with subcutaneous layer was performed in the routine fashion. Following the closure of the of the skin, bandage was applied and patient was removed to the Recovery Room in good condition.

Marsupialization of Bartholin's duct cyst

Technique

After routine prep and drape and under general anesthesia, a wedge shaped vertical incision was made in the vagina mucosa over the center of the Bartholin's gland cyst following culture of the purulent material which was present. This was performed outside the hymenal ring. Incision was made as wide as possible to enhance the postoperative patency of the stoma.

The cyst wall was then opened and drained of its remaining contents and the lining of the cyst was inverted and sutured to the vaginal mucosa on both sides with interrupted sutures of #2 _____ (delayed absorbable) material. The area was then irrigated thoroughly with Betadine and there were no drains or packs left in place.

The patient was instructed prior to pre-op anesthesia that daily sitz baths should begin on the 3rd postoperative day. The patient will be seen in the office in approximately 2–4 weeks to evaluate possible secondary fibrosis or abscess formation. A Word catheter was considered but the patient disclosed no interest in having a catheter in place for 3–4 weeks. Therefore, marsupialization was performed. The patient left the Operating Room in good condition and is in Recovery Room in good condition.

Microscopic fallopian tube reanastomosis (cornual-isthmic anastomosis)

Technique

The incision was made through the skin and down through the fascia. Peritoneum was entered with two hemostats and Metzenbaum scissors. (Document the length of fallopian tube.)

The microscope was adjusted to a magnification of approximately 10 to 20 times greater than normal so that a critical point could be reached in the anastomosis of the cornual-isthmic portions of the tube. Once the microscope had been adjusted to above the table and the patient had been placed in the supine position on operating table, her legs were then placed in the Allen stirrups. The uterus was easily exposed because of vaginal packing that had been placed into the vagina prior to the procedure. Utilizing a continuous flow of Dextran 70 from a 500 cc bag at the head of the bed on an IV pole, the end of the IV tubing continued to control the flow of irrigation throughout the microscopic surgery. Methylene blue dye was utilized during the entire procedure through the Humi dilator so that it could be determined at which point methylene blue stopped in the fallopian tube. Utilizing microscopic fine straight vascular scissors, the fallopian tube was cut in an angle until the methylene blue was noted to be spilling from the approximate portion of the fallopian tube. A #2-0 nylon monofilament suture was threaded through the tubal lumen and placed within the uterine cavity. The same procedure was carried out through the luminal side of the distal segment. The proximal obstructed end was resected and the #2-0 nylon was passed through the oviduct and out through the fimbriated end and mesosalpinx was carefully approximated to eliminate any tension at the anastomotic site. Using a _____ (#8 or #10) suture on a _____ (3-8 circle taper) needle, it was passed perpendicular to the surface of the oviductal tissue while elevating the edge of the tissue with left handed forceps while simultaneously placing the needle through the tissue avoiding any grasping of the tissue with the jaws of the forceps. Once the needle had been placed through the opposite lumen, being careful not to occlude muscularis or serosa, the suture was gently pulled with very short pulls and aligned with needle holes. This was performed to avoid damage to the tissue caused by angulation of the entry hole. The sutures were laid parallel to the oviduct and with each suture taken, the fallopian tube was pulled closely to within the area of the cornua. Hemostasis was achieved using a high frequency fine needle cautery. The two layer closure was performed using _____ (#8-0) suture. The patient was given _____ (Unasyn 3 grams) IV intraoperatively. Irrigation was performed during the entire procedure and methylene blue was injected into the Humi dilator and it was noted that the left fallopian tube spilled dye. The procedure was continued in the same manner on the opposite side.

After the entire procedure was completed the peritoneum was reapproximated with _____ (2-0) suture in a continuous manner using a nonreactive suture so that the chances of adhesive formation would be slim. Prior to closing the peritoneum, Interceed was placed over the entire operative area and between the fallopian tube and ovary. After the peritoneum was closed, muscle tissue was reapproximated with interrupted sutures of 2-0 (delayed absorbable) suture. Fascia was closed with 2-0 (delayed absorbable) suture and subcuticular layer was closed with _____ (3-0 plain) suture. The skin was reapproximated with _____ (5-0 absorbable suture) in a subcuticular fashion. $^1/_4$ inch steri-strips were placed over the incision with benzoin. Patient tolerated the procedure well. All instrumentation was removed from the vagina after proper dressing of the abdominal incision. Patient went to Recovery Room in good condition.

Myomectomy

Technique

The patient was prepped with _____ solution and draped in the standard fashion for a _____ (Pfannenstiel or vertical) incision. Surgery was continued through the subcuticular, fascial, muscle, and peritoneum with great care until the fibroid (s) was (were) located. A dilute solution of vasopressin 20 units in 60 ml of saline was injected into the cornual areas and into the lower uterine segment near each uterine artery. Approximately _____ (2–5 ml) of solution was injected into each area. Additional injections of approximately _____ (5 ml) were administered into the fibroid being excised as needed.

The incision was made into the pseudocapsule of the fibroid using a _____ (#_____ scalpel, CO2 laser, Nd: YAG laser with sapphire tip, or needle-tipped cutting cautery). The fibroid was then grasped with a towel clip. Blunt and sharp dissection were used to separate the tumor, leaving as much healthy myometrium as possible. The endometrium was avoided in its entirety.

The remaining stalk of the myoma was ligated with _____ (#2-0 delayed absorbable) suture and _____ (excised, twisted away). The crater was then irrigated thoroughly with Ringer's lactate. The "dead space" was closed with _____ (interrupted or continuous) _____ (#2-0 polyglactin or #1 delayed absorbable) suture. The serosa was then closed with a continuous _____ (#4-0) baseball stitch, using a minimum of suture exposure, thus minimizing adhesion formation.

Copious amounts of irrigation using _____ (Dextran 70, Ringer's lactate, or Mandol/normal saline) solution in the amount of _____ (150 ml) was placed in the pelvis. (This can be left to act as a floatation barrier against adhesions or _____ .) The solution was removed from the pelvis and Interceed was placed over the operative surfaces. Peritoneum was then closed with a continuous suture of _____ (#0 delayed absorbable) suture. The fascia was closed with a continuous suture of _____ (#1 delayed absorbable suture). The subcutaneous layer was closed with _____ (3-0 plain) suture. The skin was closed with _____ (5-0 Vicryl) in a continuous subcuticular stick. The incision was wiped clean with a wet lap, dry lap, then benzoin and steri-strips were applied followed by bandage. The patient's sponge, instrument, needle, and lap count were correct. She went to the Recovery Room in good condition.

Important point

- Avoid the use of vasopressin if the patient is hypertensive.

Para-aortic node dissection

Technique

The posterior peritoneum was excised and opened with Metzenbaum scissors. The incision was extended to a level above the inferior mesenteric artery and vein. A narrow _____ retractor was placed beneath the upper peritoneal margin to expose the para-aortic and para-caval regions widely.

The dissection began along the lateral margin of the left common iliac artery and continued above the inferior mesenteric vessels. Each mesenteric base of each dissected node was clamped with a vascular clip. Care was taken to avoid injury to the lumbar arteries and veins that lie behind the aorta and vena cava. Extreme caution was used while retracting the vena cava during the para-cervical node dissection so as to avoid injury to the vessel. The dissection was carried out along the lateral side of the right common iliac artery and extended on the side of the vena cava to the region above the inferior mesenteric vessels. The inferior and superior lymphatic vessels were clamped securely, excised, and ligated with _____ (#3-0 silk) tie on the tip of an _____ (Adson) clamp which provided excellent prophylaxis in preventing a subsequent lymphocyst.

(If bleeding has been troublesome during the para-aortic node dissection, a retro-peritoneal drain should be placed in the operative site and brought through the abdominal wall.) The retroperitoneum was re-approximated with a continuous _____ (2-0 delayed absorbable) suture.

Paravaginal repair

Technique

Following routine prep and drape, a Pfannenstiel incision was carried out through the skin. The incision was continued through the subcutaneous tissue and fascia so that the peritoneum could be freed from the undersurface of the rectus muscle but not entered. The recti muscles were retracted and the retropubic space was entered by incising the transversalis fascia at its attachment to the superior pubic ramus laterally until the obturator notch could be palpated while the bladder was drawn medially away from the sidewall of the pelvis. My left hand was inserted into the vagina while holding the bladder with a sponge stick. The lateral sulcus of the vagina was elevated and could be appreciated by notation of the prominent veins coursing down the lateral sulcus.

Key sutures were placed through the lateral sulcus beneath the prominent veins while elevating the lateral superior sulcus. Before releasing the needle, traction was placed on the needle holder, moving its tip toward the ischial spine. While palpating with the vaginal hand, this traction was carried backward until the external meatus of the urethra could be felt to be drawn immediately beneath the middle of the lower edge of the symphysis. The lateral pelvic wall bite was then carried out. This suture was tagged and not tied. Permanent _____ (3.0 Tycron) suture on a _____ (medium GI needle was used).

Following the key sutures that were made bilaterally, additional sutures were placed through the vaginal sulcus with its overlying pubocervical fascia and the pelvic sidewalls bilaterally. These sutures were placed at 1 cm intervals with continual interrupted placement dorsally until the last suture was placed at about 1 cm in front of the ischial spine. Once all the sutures have been placed with the most ventral suture having been placed as close as possible to the pubic ramus, at least six throws were tied for knot security in each suture.

The retropubic space was irrigated with warm Ringer's lactate solution. Hemostasis was _____ (excellent, good, etc . . . and if poor describe how it was corrected).

The fascia was closed with _____ suture. The subcutaneous tissue was closed with _____. The skin was closed with _____ .

Bandage was placed over the incision. Estimated blood loss was _____ . Sponge, lap, instrument, and needle count were _____ correct.

Posterior colporrhaphy (repair of rectocele and perineal repair)

Technique

Following proper prep and drape, the perineal skin was excised horizontally along the vaginal outlet. A midline vertical incision was initiated in the center of the mucosal edge by tunnelling beneath the posterior mucosa with Metzenbaum scissors, incising the free mucosa in the midline and extending the dissection to the apex of the vagina. In a manner similar to an anterior repair, traction was placed on the upper margin of each segment of the mucosal dissection using Allis clamps. The lower margins of the incision were held under tension with additional clamps while the mucosa was separated with Metzenbaum scissors from the underlying fascia. When the midline incision was completed, the vaginal mucosa was separated laterally from the perirectal fascia and muscle attachments by sharp dissection, taking care to avoid penetrating the thin mucosa. The lateral dissection was extended as far as possible to mobilize the perirectal fascia and to expose the medial margins of the levator ani muscles. The terminal ends of the bulbocavernosus and transverse perinei muscles were also freed from the mucosa in the lower vagina.

The perirectal fascia was then drawn over the bulging rectocele using as many vertical mattress sutures of #0 _____ (delayed absorbable) suture as were necessary to reinforce and completely close the hernial space over the rectal wall. Interrupted sutures of #1 _____ (delayed absorbable) suture were placed deeply in the margins of the levator muscles, approximating the muscles and fascia sufficiently over the lower rectal wall to produce the desired support to the perineal body and posterior vaginal wall.

After extra vaginal mucosa had been excised, the margins were closed beginning in the apex of the vagina. This was done with continuous lock stitch of 0 suture, incorporating the underlying fascia with running suture to obliterate the dead space between the vaginal wall and rectum. When the continuous mucosal suture reached the levator muscles, the deep interrupted sutures were tied. After a few supporting plication sutures were placed in the fascia and underlying muscles of the perineal body, the mucosal suture was continued over the perineum as subcuticular stitch using a small curved cutting needle. The perineal muscle sutures, including the lower margins of the bulbocavernosus and the transverse perineum muscles, gave good support to the levator hiatus and pelvic floor. The result was good. Hemostasis was judged to be excellent and the patient left the Operating Room in stable condition.

Presacral neurectomy

Author's notes

After exploratory laparotomy has been described and transcribed the following transcription should proceed.

Technique

The viscera were packed with wet lap packs and _____ retractor was used to expose the sacral promontory. The retroperitoneal space was dissected using a vertical incision. Adventitia and adipose tissue along the retroperitoneal fat area was dissected using hemoclips and Metzenbaum scissors. Care was taken to expose both bilateral ureters which passed over the aortic bifurcation on both sides and these were moved out of the operative field being careful not to denude any blood supply or tissue from around the edges of the ureters. Bleeding was brought to hemostasis with hemoclips as the adventitia was dissected away from the presacral nerve plexus. The nerve plexus was elevated with right angle forceps and tied with a free tie along the superior edge and along the superior inferior edge with another pair of right angle forceps. Free tie was brought around the posterior inferior edge of the presacral nerve plexus and this was also tied with 0- _____ (delayed absorbable) suture.

After being tied at the superior and inferior borders, the presacral nerve plexus was excised and removed from the retroperitoneal space. Hemostasis was judged to be adequate and the retroperitoneal space and adventitia was closed with 2-0 _____ (chromic or delayed absorbable) in a continuous suture. _____ (Interceed) was placed over this portion of the surgery. After packs had been removed and viscera replaced back into the anatomical position, _____ Interceed was placed under the peritoneal closure using 2-0 _____ (delayed absorbable) suture, thereby decreasing the chance of any postoperative adhesions. The fascia was closed in a continuous suture of #0 _____ (delayed absorbable) suture. The skin was closed with _____ (skin staples). Bandage was applied. Patient tolerated the procedure very well.

Sacrospinous ligament fixation

Technique

After routine prep and drape, ligament fixation was started as the posterior vaginal wall was exposed and incised to its full thickness up to the apex through the endopelvic fascia until the rectovaginal space was entered. This was performed with Metzenbaum scissors and single-layer sponges, performed both sharply and bluntly.

The peritoneum was then resected with the posterior vaginal mucosa. The patient's right rectovaginal space was then dissected bluntly to the level of the ischial spines, and the right descending rectal pillar was perforated bluntly and sharply so that the ischial spines and sacrospinous/coccygeal complex could be adequately visualized. The perirectal space was entered. Additional blunt sharp dissection was performed until the ischial spine and sacrospinous ligament/coccygeus muscle complex were palpated and visually identified. Under direct visualization and using a Miya hook ligature carrier to the sacrospinous ligaments, two #2 _____ (Prolene) sutures were placed through the sacrospinous/coccygeus ligament complex, approximately 2–3 cm medial to the ischial spine. After the sutures were placed in the sacrospinous/coccygeus muscle complex and through the ligament, the correctness of their placement was tested by pulling on them firmly. These sutures were then tagged.

The sacrospinous fixation was completed utilizing a pulley and a safety stitch. The pulley stitch was placed by throwing a half-knot through the suture that was taken in the posterior vaginal apex. When the end of the suture attached to the pulley stitch was held with moderate tension, the other end of the suture was drawn out allowing the apex to be drawn snugly against the sacrospinous/coccygeal complex. The safety stitch was then tied in normal fashion. The vagina was checked and found to be slightly deviated to the right. A few 2-0 _____ (chromic) sutures were placed over the area of ligament fixation and interlocked in a continuous fashion to completely close the vagina. The vagina was noted to be seen in the normal anatomical position with slight deviation to the right, and the vagina was thoroughly irrigated with a _____ (normal saline cefamandole solution), dried, then packed with _____ (iodoform) packing. Transurethral catheter was left to gravity. The patient tolerated the procedure well and went to the Recovery Room in good condition.

Author's notes

(1) Usually this procedure requires additional combination procedures such as the following transcription, see A&P with Enterocele Repair.

(2) The Shutt Suture Punch System, an orthopedic instrument, has been shown to allow safe and rapid placement and retrieval of suture into the sacrospinous ligament for suspension of the vagina. The technique is described by T. R. Sharp in The Journal of the American College of Obstetricians and Gynecologists, Volume 82, p. 893, 1993.

Sacrospinous ligament fixation with anterior and posterior colporrhaphy and with complete repair of vaginal vault

Technique

The patient was prepped and draped in the usual manner, and a catheter was placed. A weighted speculum was placed into the vagina, and the vaginal vault prolapse was spontaneously noted to be protruding out of the introitus. Bulging cystocele, rectocele, and enterocele could be noted. The anterior colporrhaphy was performed first with the entire length of the anterior vaginal wall dissected after Neo-Synephrine injection. This was performed with Metzenbaum scissors and Allis clamps in the routine manner, pushing the cystocele away from the vaginal mucosa with a single layer of gauze sponge.

After the cystocele had been fully dissected away from the vaginal mucosa the retropubic urethral ligaments were plicated in a manner which resituated the posterior urethral vesicle angle retropubically by pulling #1 _____ (chromic) sutures underneath the urethra. The remaining endopelvic fascia was then plicated in the midline, reducing the cystocele using interrupted locking sutures on #1 _____ . The vaginal mucosa was trimmed away, and the vaginal mucosa was then reapproximated with 2-0 _____ in the usual manner.

Ligament fixation was then started as the posterior vaginal wall was exposed and incised to its full thickness up to the apex through the endopelvic fascia until the rectovaginal space was entered. This was performed with Metzenbaum scissors and single-layer sponges, performed both sharply and bluntly. The enterocele sac was grasped with a Kelly clamp and opened into the peritoneum. The ureters were located, palpated, and avoided. The peritoneum was repaired with a highly placed purse-string suture in the routine manner.

The peritoneum was then resected with the posterior vaginal mucosa. The patient's right rectovaginal space was then dissected bluntly to the level of the ischial spines, and the right descending rectal pillar was perforated bluntly and sharply so that the ischial

139

spines and sacrospinous/coccygeal complex could be adequately visualized. The perirectal space was entered. Additional blunt sharp dissection was performed until the ischial spine and sacrospinous ligament/coccygeus muscle complex were palpated and visually identified. Under direct visualization and using a Miya hook ligature carrier to the sacrospinous ligaments, two #2 _____ (Prolene) sutures were placed through the sacrospinous/ coccygeus ligament complex, approximately 2–3 cm medial to the ischial spine. After the sutures were placed in the sacrospinous/ coccygeus muscle complex and through the ligament, the correctness of their placement was tested by pulling on them firmly. These sutures were then tagged.

The rectocele was then repaired by performing an excision along the peritoneal skin, and then horizontally along the vaginal outlet. Midline vertical incision was initiated in the center of the mucosal edge by tunnelling beneath the posterior mucosa with Metzenbaum scissors and incising the free mucosa in the midline and extending the dissection of the apex to the vagina.

In a manner similar to the anterior repair, traction was placed on the upper margin of each segment of mucosal dissection using Allis clamps. The lower margins of the incisions were held under tension with additional clamps while the mucosa was separated with Metzenbaum scissors from the underlying fascia. When the midline incision was completed, the vaginal mucosa was separated laterally from the perineal fascia and muscle attachments by sharp dissection, taking care to avoid penetrating the mucosa. The lateral dissection was extended as far as possible to mobilize the perirectal fascia and expose the medial margins of the levator and muscles. These were already exposed from the dissection in the rectovaginal space during the Miya hook suspension. The terminal ends of the bulbocavernosus and transverse perineal muscles were also freed from the mucosa and the lower vagina. The perirectal fascia was then drawn over the bulging rectocele, using as many vertical mattress sutures of #0 _____ (delayed absorbable) sutures as were necessary to reinforce and completely close the hernial space of the rectal wall. Interrupted sutures of #1 _____ (delayed absorbable) suture were placed deeply in the margin of the levator muscles, approximating the muscles and fascia sufficiently over the lower rectal wall to produce the desired support for the perineal body and posterior vaginal wall. After the extravaginal mucosa had been excised, the margins were closed, beginning at the apex of the vagina. This was performed with continuous lock-suture of 0-suture incorporating the underlying fascia and running suture to obliterate the dead space between the vagina and rectum. When the continuous mucosal sutures were completed and the levator muscles reached, the deep interrupted sutures were tied. After a few supporting plication sutures were placed in the fascia and underlying muscles of the perineal body, the mucosal suture was continued over the perineum as a subcuticular stitch using a small, curved cutting needle. The perineal muscle sutures including the lower margins of the bulbocavernosus and transverse perinei muscles, gave good support to the levator hiatus and pelvic floor. The result was good. Hemostasis was judged to be excellent.

The sacrospinous fixation was completed utilizing a pulley and a safety stitch. The pulley stitch was placed by throwing a halfknot through the suture that was taken in the posterior vaginal apex. When the end of the suture attached to the pulley stitch was held with moderate tension, the other end of the suture was drawn out allowing the apex to be drawn snugly against the sacrospinous/coccygeal complex. The safety stitch was then tied in normal fashion. The vagina was checked and found to be slightly deviated to the right. A few 2-0 _____ (chromic) sutures were placed over the area of ligament fixation and interlocked in a continuous fashion to completely close the vagina. The vagina was noted to be seen in the normal anatomical position with slight deviation to the right, and the vagina was thoroughly irrigated with a _____ (normal saline/cefamandole solution), dried, then packed with _____ (iodoform) packing. Transurethral catheter was left to gravity. The patient tolerated the procedure well and went to the Recovery Room in good condition.

Author's note

The Shutt Suture Punch System, an orthopedic instrument, has been shown to allow safe and rapid placement and retrieval of suture into the sacrospinous ligament for suspension of the vagina. This technique is described by T.R. Sharp in The Journal of the American College of Obstetricians and Gynecologists, Volume 82, p. 893, 1993.

Salpingectomy

Technique

After the patient had been placed in the supine position and routine prep and drape had been performed, the incision was made and was carried down through the subcutaneous fat to the fascia. Hemostasis was obtained utilizing hemostats and the electrocautery. The fascia was incised with the scalpel blade and extended with Mayo scissors. Midline was opened between the two rectus sheaths and the peritoneum was picked up with two hemostats and with the scalpel blade. The peritoneum was then extended with the Metzenbaum scissors and _____ (O'Sullivan or Balfour) retractor was placed in the peritoneal cavity. Necessary exposure was obtained and _____ (describe the findings).

The above findings being noted, neither salpingotomy, manual expression, or segmental resection could be performed. The affected fallopian tube was elevated and the mesosalpinx were clamped with a succession of Kelly clamps at the serosa of the tube, as close as possible to the tube. The tube was then excised by cutting a small myometrial wedge at the uterine cornu. Figure of eight sutures of 0 _____ (delayed absorbable) material was used to close the myometrium at the site of the wedge resection. The mesosalpinx was closed with interrupted sutures of 0 _____ (delayed absorbable) suture. Complete hemostasis was noted. The fundus was held forward and the round and broad ligaments were sutured over the uterine cornu in a modified Coffey technique accomplishing complete peritonealization. Mattress sutures anchored the broad ligament to the uterus. A 0 _____ (delayed absorbable) suture was used to penetrate the broad ligament from its anterior surface just below the round ligaments, approximately 2–3 cm from the cornua. The second bite was taken into the fundus of the uterus, slightly posterior and superior to the uterine incision. The suture was then placed through the posterior aspect of the broad ligament, approximately 1 cm lateral to the previous suture. After this suture was tied, the cornual incision in the mesosalpinx was peritonealized. There was no excessive tension on this suture and supporting sutures were placed in the myometrium and the round ligament to be certain that peritonealization would remain in place. Hemostasis was judged to be excellent.

After thorough irrigation of the peritoneal cavity, Kelly clamps were used on the edges of the peritoneum so as to close the peritoneum in a continuous suture of 2-0 _____ . Three point suturing was used to avert the cut peritoneal edges and make the intraperitoneal suture line as smooth as possible. Fascial edges were approximated following reapproximation of the rectus sheath with a single suture of #1 _____ in a continuous fashion. Subcutaneous layer was irrigated thoroughly and then approximated with continuous sutures of 3-0 _____ on a _____ needle. The skin was reapproximated in the routine fashion and the patient left the Operating Room in stable condition.

Salpingotomy (linear)

Technique

(Describe the laparotomy portion and findings.) The affected fallopian tube was exposed, elevated and stabilized. A linear incision was made with _____ (scalpel or laser) over the distended segment of the tube. The incision was extended through the antimesenteric wall until entry was made into the lumen of the distended ova duct. Gentle pressure was then exerted from the opposite side of the fallopian tube. The products of gestation were gently expressed from the lumen. Gentle traction with forceps without teeth and gentle suction were used but care was taken to avoid trauma to the mucosa. Remaining fragments of the anchoring trophoblast were removed by profuse irrigation of the lumen with warm Ringer's lactate solution. Small tubal vessels were easily identified while the fallopian tube was being irrigated and complete hemostasis to tubal mucosa was brought into effect utilizing an ophthalmological cautery.

Mucosal margins were then closed with interrupted sutures of 7-0 _____ (delayed absorbable) suture making sure that only the serosa and muscularis were approximated without undue tension. Care was taken to ensure that no suture material was retained on the mucosal surface. After hemostasis was judged to be adequate, the abdomen was explored for extra blood clots and these were all removed. Proper irrigation was performed and the peritoneum was closed along the posterior rectus sheath with a continuous suture of 2-0 _____ suture. Three point suture was used to avert cut peritoneal edges to make the intraperitoneal suture line as smooth as possible. The bilateral rectus sheath muscles were reapproximated with interrupted _____ sutures. The fascia was then reapproximated with single sutures of #1 _____ in a continuous fashion. The subcutaneous fat was reapproximated with 3-0 _____ . The skin was then reapproximated and bandage was applied. The patient was removed to the Recovery Room in stable condition.

Author's notes

When closing the mucosal margins, it is optional to use no suture, thus leaving the tube open.

Sterilization procedures

Overview

As important as operative transcription, other documentation in regards to sterilization is very important. During history, operative, or discharge notes it might be useful as a guideline to document the following:

(1) The patient understands that she will be permanently unable to bear children, even though the success rate of subsequent reversal might be high.

(2) She understands that effectiveness is not guaranteed and that a failure rate of 5 per 1000 procedures are known to occur with the commonly performed procedures.

(3) Operative and anesthetic complications such as hemorrhage, bowel, ureteral, and bladder damage have been explained to the patient and she understands including the possibility of death (1 out of 30,000 procedures).

(4) Explanation of the various methods available are understood by the patient and she has chosen _____ . (Document if she was given a pamphlet or if she was allowed to view a video demonstrating the various methods.)

(5) The patient has had pointed out to her that technical problems or complications can turn a laparoscopy into laparotomy (particularly mention this in conjunction with patients that may have had prior abdominal or pelvic surgery).

(6) Be sure the consent is clear, specific, and spells out *permanent* results but that *failure is possible*.

(7) Perform the surgery early in the patient's cycle, perform a pregnancy test, and/or inform the patient about the possibility of pregnancy at the time of interval sterilization. Advise and document that the patient understands the possibility of ectopic pregnancy following tubal ligation (half the pregnancies that follow tubal ligation are ectopic) and that she needs to report any symptoms of pregnancy!

Important points

- Most failures with clips occur when the clip is placed too distal on the tube or at oblique angles to the axis of the tube. Make certain that the Hulka clip is within 3 cm of the uterus but not too close either in that at least 3 cm of isthmus next to the uterus will minimize the chance of uteroperitoneal fistual and, in turn, an ectopic pregnancy.

- A Falope ring can fail if not enough tube is drawn into the ring, so make certain there is an adequate loop of tube above the band.

- If video equipment is available for videolaparoscopic documentation, use it. Of course, this medical-legal documentation can backfire in court if the technique is documented as poor and the patient is pregnant. Video would most definitely be helpful if a repeat procedure is necessary.

- Avoid using single rather than double ligatures. Avoid techniques such as the Madlener (not described in this book because of its high failure rate).

- If colpotomy is performed, use prophylactic antibiotics or simply avoid this method because tubal occlusion performed through the vagina is associated with a higher rate of pelvic abscess and other complications.

- Be familiar with the institutional bipolar equipment. Use waveform rather than coagulation or blended form. Use a power setting of at least 25 watts. Coagulate at least 3 cm of tube and/or transect the tube to decrease the possibility of pregnancy.

- Pathology specimens are not necessary to prove occlusion and may increase the possibility of complications but if a pathology report is ordered, make certain that it is given full attention. A hysterosalpingogram might be helpful post-operatively to document tubal occlusion if a full lumen has not been documented by the pathologist.

HYSTEROSCOPIC SILICONE PLUG TECHNIQUE

Technique

Bimanual vaginal examination was performed so that the size of the uterus and orientation of the uterine corpus in relation to the cervix was determined.

After routine scrubbing, gloving, prepping, and draping – a speculum was inserted and the cervix and vagina were again disinfected over a wide area. (If paracervical anesthesia is used – describe here.) The optical assembly was mounted on the instrument with care not to soil the optics and sleeves. Initially, the _____ flow rate was set at _____ . (For CO_2 this rate is 75 ml/min but Dextran 70 is the distention medium currently being used in the Netherlands.)

A single tooth tenaculum was used to grasp the anterior lip of the cervix and traction with the left hand corrected for proper vaginal axis.

The end of the hysteroscope was inserted so as to examine the plicae palmate which appeared _____ (essentially normal if so). The lens then came in contact with the internal os and after approximately 15-20 seconds, the _____ (CO_2) pressure dilated the orifice and the hysteroscope was then advanced to the center of the orifice. The instrument was then advanced into the uterine cavity without injury or complication.

Flow rate of _____ (30 ml/min for CO_2) was then adjusted for the remainder of the procedure. The uterine cavity was explored in a systematic manner, examining the anterior, posterior, side walls, fundus and cornua. (Describe any significant findings or state that all was normal in that PID is a contraindication for this procedure.)

The disposable catheter from the Ovabloc kit was placed through the operative channel of the hysteroscope and the catheter was placed into the ostium of the right fallopian tube. The radiopaque silicone monomer was then injected into the right fallopian tube until complete plugging was apparent. The same procedure was performed on the left tube. Examination revealed no perforation of the uterine fundus and no apparent injury to any pelvic organs.

Instrumentation was removed from the cervix and vagina. The patient was in stable condition. The patient was advised to undergo pelvic X-ray in three months prior to coitus without contraception. She was alert and understood these instructions prior to discharge.

Author's notes

Determine that the patient is in the first half of her menstrual cycle (this is the best time to perform hysteroscopy in that the uterine mucosa is thin and the internal cervical os is easier to pass and there is no risk of pregnancy).

This procedure has not been FDA approved except for research use as a permanent method, as of publication of this book. It is not recommended until all study results in regards to the use of the silicone catalytic polymerization in situ has been fully evaluated. Although this method is promising for the future, since it is investigational, this point should certainly be explained to the patient and all aspects documented in full detail if this technique is used at this time.

IRVING STERILIZATION

Technique

Following routine prep, drape, and _____ (laparotomy or minilap), the right fallopian tube was located and doubly ligated with #2-0 _____ approximately 3 cm from the uterine cornu and then severed. The sutures on the proximal end of the tube were left long. This tubal stump was then dissected free from the mesosalpinx and mobilized. A small nick was made in the serosa on the posterior surface of the uterus near the cornu in as avascular an area as could be found and musculature was penetrated with mosquito clamp for approximately 1 cm and with the clamp spread sufficiently to admit the tube. The fallopian tube and one of the ligatures attached to the tubal stump was threaded with a round needle. Guided by a groove director, the needle was thrust to the bottom of the pocket created by the mosquito clamp and carried out to the uterine surface. The other suture attached to the tubal stump was treated in a similar manner, bringing it to the surface of the uterus about 1 cm from the first suture. Traction was exerted on the sutures and tubal stump was buried in the uterine musculature. The sutures were then tied together and a suture of fine _____ was used to close the edges of the pocket more tightly around the buried tube.

The same procedure was performed on the left fallopian tube in that it was doubly ligated with #2-0 _____ approximately 3 cm from the uterine cornu and then severed. The sutures of the proximal end of the fallopian tube were left long and this tubal stump was then dissected free from the mesosalpinx and mobilized. A small incision was made in the serosa on the posterior surface of the uterus near the cornu in an avascular area and the musculature was penetrated with mosquito clamp for about 1 cm. With the clamp spread sufficiently to admit the fallopian tube, one of the ligatures attached to the tube was threaded with a round needle and was guided by a groove director and the needle was thrust to the bottom of the pocket created by the mosquito clamp and carried out to the uterine surface. The other suture attached to the tubal stump was treated in similar manner, bringing it to the surface of the uterus about 1 cm from the first suture. Traction was exerted on the sutures and the tubal stump was buried in the uterine musculature. The sutures were then tied together and suture of fine _____ was used to close the edges of the pocket more tightly about the tube.

At the completion of the sterilization, hemostasis was found to be excellent and the remainder of the operation was performed in the routine manner. Describe closure.

Author's notes

A modified Irving operation was performed and transcribed secondary to knowledge that according to the classical Irving's original description of the operation, the ligated end of the distal portion of the fallopian tube was buried beneath the leaves of the broad ligament. The burying of this end of the tube is presently considered to be optional because it gives a neat appearance and adds nothing to the effectiveness of the sterilization. Furthermore, it adds a slightly more dangerous step to the procedure in that a blood vessel may be nicked occasionally during this step.

KROENER METHOD

Author's note

Type of incision must be described in that minilaparotomy, laparotomy, or even colpotomy may be performed during this method of sterilization.

Technique

Following exposure of the fimbriated end of the oviduct into the operative field, the fallopian tube was grasped with a Babcock clamp. The mesosalpinx and outer third of the fallopian tube were clamped, doubly ligated with #2 absorbable sutures twice and excised to remove the entire fimbriated end of the fallopian tube. The outer third of the fallopian tube was grasped with a Heaney clamp, and the initial ligature was a free tie to secure the blood vessels in the mesosalpinx. A transfixing ligature through the wall of the fallopian tube was placed between the Heaney clamp and the initial ligature to completely secure the collateral circulation and to occlude the lumen of the oviduct. The fimbriated end of the tube was then excised with Metzenbaum scissors between the clamp and the outer ligature. Following the excision of the fimbria and small segment of the ampullary portion of the fallopian tube, it was noted that the entire functional component of the oviduct was completely removed.

The same was performed on both fallopian tubes. Hemostasis was judged to be excellent. The incision was reapproximated in the routine fashion. All instrument counts, lap counts, and sponge counts were correct. Estimated blood loss was _____ . The patient tolerated the procedure well and went to the Recovery Room in good condition.

LAPAROSCOPIC STERILIZATION TECHNIQUES – BILATERAL PARTIAL SALPINGECTOMY

Technique

The patient was prepped with solution and draped in the lithotomy position with special attention to the area of the umbilicus and cervix. Weighted speculum was placed into the vagina so as to expose the cervix. A _____ tenaculum was placed into the cervix to enable the uterus to be manipulated. The weighted speculum was removed and the bladder was emptied with a catheter. Gloves were then changed prior to abdominal incision.

A small subumbilical incision was performed and _____ Verres needle was placed into the incision and checked by the syringe, the hanging drop, the bubble, and the gas pressure register methods. All methods indicated proper placement of the needle.

Pneumoperitoneum of approximately 3 liters of CO_2 was established then _____ trocar was properly inserted into the abdomen. The sound of escaping gas confirmed proper location in the abdomen as the trocar was removed from the sleeve.

Fiberoptics (and videocamera if available) were connected to the laparoscope and this was inserted through the sleeve under _____ (direct or video) laparoscopic visualization. Trendelenburg position was increased and approximately 1–1.5 liters more of CO_2 gas was allowed into the abdomen to displace the viscera, so as to easily visualize the pelvic organs. (Describe the findings.)

Laparoscopic flat duckbill bipolar forceps were brought into contact with the right fallopian tube and mesosalpinx. Coagulation and avulsion of the tube was performed for approximately 10 seconds over a distal, midportion and proximal area of the middle one-third of the fallopian tube. The cauterized segment of the tube and mesosalpinx were then transected twice with a pair of laparoscopic hook scissors. The middle portion of this cauterized segment was removed. Hemostasis was judged to be excellent during the entire procedure. The exact same procedure was performed on the opposite left fallopian tube. Both fallopian tubes were observed to be adequately cauterized and transected. The procedure was discontinued and the abdomen was inspected. Hemostasis was excellent. There was no apparent injury to any bladder, bowel, vessels, or other visceral structures. The CO_2 was released from the abdominal cavity. All instrumentation was removed from the abdomen. The subumbilical incision was reapproximated with a figure-of-eight suture utilizing 3-0 _____ suture. Neosporin and bandaid were applied to the incision. All instrumentation was removed from the vagina and the patient went to the Recovery Room in excellent condition.

LAPAROSCOPIC STERILIZATION TECHNIQUES – CAUTERIZATION AND TRANSECTION OF THE FALLOPIAN TUBES

Technique

The patient was prepped and draped in the usual manner and placed in the modified lithotomy position with the legs at 45 degree angle axis to the table. After assuring that her buttocks extended over the edge of the operating table, the table was tilted to approximately 15 degrees of Trendelenburg's position to help the peritoneum displace the intestines out of the pelvis. With the patient properly positioned on the table, bimanual examination and vaginal cleansing was performed. The abdominal wall was scrubbed with and painted with antiseptic solution with special attention directed around the umbilicus. The patient's bladder was emptied by catheter and vaginal retractor was inserted and the anterior lip of the cervix was grasped with _____ tenaculum and inserted into the uterine cavity for uterine manipulation.

The outer surgical gloves were removed and with underlying surgical gloves in place, attention was focused on the abdominal cavity. A 2 mm skin incision was made in the lower margin of the umbilicus. A large bore Verres needle was placed into the incision and inserted through the incision and passed down to the fascia while counter traction was applied by means of surgeon and assistant pressure on the skin at 5 o'clock and 7 o'clock of the incision. A quick, short plunge of the needle through the abdominal fascia and peritoneum directed toward the center of the uterus was performed and the needle was tested to determine whether it had been properly placed. Gas pressure registered by the CO_2 pneumoperitoneum was noted not to be elevated and then attachment of the gas tubing was performed and approximately 3 liters of gas was allowed to form a pneumoperitoneum. With the pneumoperitoneum established, the needle was withdrawn and umbilical incision was enlarged from 2 mm to approximately 1 cm.

A laparoscopic trocar and sleeve were inserted through the incision with a twisting motion and utilizing the lifted abdomen with the assistant's hand. The trocar was inserted as far as the rectus fascia. The trocar and sleeve were then angled to a point slightly toward the pelvis and a short, quick, stabbing motion was used to penetrate the rectus fascia and peritoneum all at once. The trocar was withdrawn from its sleeve and the trumpet valve on the sleeve was depressed slightly so as to listen for the sound of gas escaping for the pneumoperitoneum. This sound confirmed that the trocar sleeve was properly located and then this was shut to ensure that the gas would no longer escape. A fiberoptic light cable was now connected to the laparoscope and the light turned on. Laparoscope was gently inserted into the trocar sleeve while watching through the eyepiece. Laparoscope was inserted in an angle to the abdomen approximately 15–20 degrees and the laparoscope was then advanced into the pelvis to identify the structures there. The gas hose was then connected to the gas port on the sleeve. A small amount of gas (approximately 1–1.5 liters) was allowed to flow into the abdomen to better displace the intestines out of the pelvis. The pelvis was then thoroughly inspected for visible gynecological abnormalities. (Describe findings.)

Following the laparoscopic examination, the uterus was manipulated to bring the fallopian tube on the right into view. The forceps handle was closed and this compressed the fallopian tube and simultaneously brought the flat, duckbill portion of the tips in contact with the mesosalpinx. After the first burn and avulsion of the tube, the second burn was applied to the proximal stump. The electric current was applied for approximately 10 seconds. The cauterized segment of the tube and mesosalpinx were transected then with a pair of hook scissors. Hemostasis was judged to be excellent. The same was performed on the opposite fallopian tube. After both fallopian tubes were observed to be very adequately transected, the procedure was discontinued and the CO_2 gas was released from the abdominal cavity.

All instrumentation was removed from the abdomen. After

reapproximation of the incision with 3-0 _____ , a bandaid was applied to the area and the instruments were removed from the vagina. The patient was removed to the Recovery Room in excellent condition.

LAPAROSCOPIC STERILIZATION TECHNIQUES – SPRING-LOADED CLIP OR HULKA TECHNIQUE

Technique

The patient was prepped and draped in the usual manner and placed in the modified lithotomy position with the legs at 45 degree angle axis to the table. After assuring that her buttocks extended over the edge of the operating table, the table was tilted to approximately 15 degrees of Trendelenburg's position to help the peritoneum displace the intestines out of the pelvis. With the patient properly positioned on the table, bimanual examination and vaginal cleansing was performed. The abdominal wall was scrubbed with _____ and painted with antiseptic solution with special attention directed around the umbilicus. The patient's bladder was emptied by catheter and vaginal retractor was inserted and the anterior lip of the cervix was grasped with _____ tenaculum and inserted into the uterine cavity for uterine manipulation. The outer surgical gloves were removed and with underlying surgical gloves in place, attention was focused on the abdominal cavity. A 2 mm skin incision was made in the lower margin of the umbilicus. A large bore _____ Verres needle was placed into the incision and inserted through the incision and passed down to the fascia while counter traction was applied by means of surgeon and assistant pressure on the skin at 5 o'clock and 7 o'clock of the incision. A quick, short plunge of the needle through the abdominal fascia and peritoneum directed toward the center of the uterus was performed and the needle was tested to determine whether it had been properly placed. The _____ test was utilized to determine proper placement. (Describe results of test.) Gas pressure registered by the CO_2 pneumoperitoneum was noted not to be elevated and then attachment of the gas tubing was performed and approximately 3 liters of gas was allowed to form a pneumoperitoneum. With the pneumoperitoneum established, the needle was withdrawn and umbilical incision was enlarged from 2 mm to approximately 1 cm. A laparoscopic _____ trocar and sleeve were inserted through the incision with a twisting motion and utilizing the lifted abdomen with the assistant's hand. The trocar was inserted as far as the rectus fascia. The trocar and sleeve were then angled to a point slightly toward the pelvis and a short, quick, stabbing motion was used to penetrate the rectus fascia and peritoneum all at once. The trocar was withdrawn from its sleeve and the trumpet valve on the sleeve was depressed slightly so as to listen for the sound of gas escaping for the pneumoperitoneum. This sound confirmed that the trocar sleeve was properly located and then this was shut to ensure that the gas would no longer escape. A fiberoptic light cable was now connected to the laparoscope and the light turned on. (Describe if video camera is attached.) Laparoscope was gently inserted into the trocar sleeve while watching through the eyepiece (or while watching the video screen if videolaparoscopy is used). Laparoscope was inserted in an angle to the abdomen approximately 15–20 degrees and the laparoscope was then advanced into the pelvis to identify the structures there. The gas hose was then connected to the gas port on the sleeve. A small amount of gas (approximately 1–1.5 liters) was allowed to flow into the abdomen to better displace the intestines out of the pelvis. The pelvis was then thoroughly inspected for visible gynecological abnormalities. (Describe any abnormalities.)

Following the placement of laparoscopic instruments, the spring loaded clip consisting of two small serrated Silastic jaws held together by the metal clip with the teeth at the end of the jaws which locked the clip into place, was attached to the fallopian tube with applicator. This was performed on the right fallopian tube. The same application was performed on the left tube as was performed on the right tube. Following completion of the application, the instrumentation was removed from the abdomen and release of the gas from the abdomen was performed. The incision was reapproximated with 3-0 chromic in the routine fashion and the instruments were also removed from the vagina. The patient went to the Recovery Room in good condition. Blood loss was mininal. Counts were correct.

Author's notes

(1)   Although the failure rate with this method (Clip or Hulka) is 2%, and seems somewhat higher than with other laparoscopic sterilization methods, the damage to the tube is felt to be less and for this reason this was used on this patient since she may wish to have reversal of sterilization in the future (it might be preferable to add this type comment either in the history or operative transcription to this effect).

(2)   With all laparoscopic techniques performed under *local anesthesia*, it is necessary to transcribe the type of anesthetic injected and method used prior to the umbilical skin incision.

LAPAROSCOPIC STERILIZATION TECHNIQUES – FALOPE RING (YOON OR SILASTIC BAND TECHNIQUE)

Technique

The patient was prepped and draped in the usual manner and placed in the modified lithotomy position with the legs at 45 degree angle axis to the table. After assuring that her buttocks extended over the edge of the operating table, the table was tilted to approximately 15 degrees of Trendelenburg's position to help the peritoneum displace the intestines out of the pelvis. With the patient properly positioned on the table, bimanual examination and vaginal cleansing was performed. The abdominal wall was scrubbed with _____ and painted with antiseptic solution with special attention directed around the umbilicus. The patient's bladder was emptied by catheter and vaginal retractor was inserted and the anterior lip of the cervix was grasped with _____ tenaculum and inserted into the uterine cavity for manipulation. The outer surgical gloves were removed and with underlying surgical gloves in place, attention was focused on the abdominal cavity. A 2 mm skin incision was made in the lower margin of the umbilicus. A large bore _____ needle was placed into the incision and inserted through the incision and passed down to the fascia while counter traction was applied by means of surgeon and assistant pressure on the skin at 5 o'clock and 7 o'clock of the incision. A quick, short plunge of the needle through the abdominal fascia and peritoneum directed toward the center of the uterus was performed and the needle was tested to determine whether it had been properly placed. The test was utilized to determine proper placement. (Describe the results of the test.)

Gas pressure registered by the CO_2 pneumoperitoneum was noted not to be elevated and then attachment of the gas tubing was performed and approximately 3 liters of gas was allowed to form a pneumoperitoneum. With the pneumoperitoneum established, the needle was withdrawn and umbilical incision was enlarged from 2 mm to approximately 1 cm.

A laparoscopic trocar and sleeve were inserted through the incision with a twisting motion and utilizing the lifted abdomen with the assistant's hand. The trocar was inserted as far as the rectus fascia. The trocar and sleeve were then angled to a point slightly toward the pelvis and a short, quick, stabbing motion was used to penetrate the rectus fascia and peritoneum all at once. The trocar was withdrawn from its sleeve and the trumpet valve on the sleeve was depressed slightly so as to listen for the sound of gas escaping for the pneumoperitoneum. This sound confirmed that the trocar sleeve was properly located and then this was shut to ensure that the gas would no longer escape. A fiberoptic light cable was now connected to the laparoscope and the light turned on. Laparoscope was gently inserted into the trocar sleeve while watching through the eyepiece. Laparoscope was inserted in an angle to the abdomen approximately 15–20 degrees and the laparoscope was then advanced into the pelvis to identify the structures there. The gas hose was then connected to the gas port on the sleeve. A small amount of gas (approximately 1–1.5 liters) was allowed to flow into the abdomen to better displace the intestines out of the pelvis. The pelvis was then thoroughly inspected for visible gynecological abnormalities. (Describe findings.)

Following the completion of the placement of the laparoscopic instruments, the specially equipped laparoscope which was loaded with Silastic band (Falope ring) was inserted in standard fashion. *(Some of the newer models can accommodate two rings simultaneously making it possible to enable the operator to apply both rings to each tube without having to bring the scope back out through the sleeve to reload. Some of the newer versions also have canals that allow optional application of local anesthetic that may temporarily decrease postoperative discomfort. If this anesthetic is applied to the tube – it should be transcribed here.)* The tongs at the band applicator were then extended and the right fallopian tube was grasped at the ampullo-isthmic junction and brought into the applicator. The band was pushed over a knuckle of the tube and then the tongs were released and the tube was dropped into the cul-de-sac. The left fallopian tube was treated in the same manner as the right. Instrumentation was removed from the abdomen. As much CO_2 was removed at this time as possible. Closure of the incision was performed with 3-0 _____ . Vaginal instrumentation was removed and the patient tolerated the procedure well.

Author's notes

If the local anesthesia is applied for the aid in relief of postoperative pain after tubal sterilization with Falope rings, then insert "each fallopian tube was sprayed with 5 cc of 0.5% bupivacaine".

Footnote

The mesosalpinx of each tube can also be injected with 3-5 cc of 0.5% bupivacaine after application of the rings but this method can increase the possibility of bleeding and has not been demonstrated significantly to reduce pain or shorten recovery room stays over the "spray" method.

Reference

Borgatta; American Journal of GYN Health, VOL. 5, No. 1 Jan/ Feb 1991.

MINI-LAP POMEROY STERILIZATION

Technique

Following the placement of the patient in the supine position and after proper prep and drape, a small mini-lap incision was made transversely over the suprapubic area and carried down to the subcutaneous fascia. Fascia was entered with scalpel blade and extended with Mayo scissors and the peritoneum was grasped with 2 hemostats and entered with Metzenbaum scissors. The peritoneum was extended with Metzenbaum scissors and the uterus was located with the surgeon's fingers.

Following the location of the uterus, the fallopian tube was grasped with Babcock clamp and delivered. After identification of the fimbria of the right fallopian tube, a midportion of the right fallopian tube was held up and ligated twice with a #2 absorbable suture. The loop was then cut off with Metzenbaum scissors and hemostasis was brought into effect with the electrocautery. The fallopian tube was placed back into the peritoneum and the left fallopian tube was located with the surgeon's finger and delivered through the incision with Babcock clamp around the midportion of the fallopian tube. After identification of the fimbriated end, the loop was held up and it was ligated twice with an absorbable #2 plain suture. The loop was then cut off with the Metzenbaum scissors and hemostasis was brought into effect. The bisected tube was then placed back into the peritoneum and both portions of fallopian tube were handed off to the surgical scrub nurse.

Peritoneum was then reapproximated with a continuous absorbable suture and the fascia was reapproximated with # 2-0 _____ continuous suture. The subcutaneous tissue was closed with _____ suture.

A subcuticular suture was used in a continuous fashion

utilizing #5-0 _____ . The patient tolerated the procedure well and the incisional area was applied with bandage. The patient went to the Recovery Room in good condition. Counts were correct and blood loss minimal.

POSTPARTUM POMEROY STERILIZATION

Technique

Following delivery, the patient was prepared for surgery in the routine manner. A small subumbilical incision was performed and the peritoneum easily entered. The fundus of the uterus was easily located with the surgeon's fingers through the incision and the fallopian tube was swept into view so that the midportion of the tube could be grasped with Babcock clamps and delivered. As the loop was held up, the fallopian tube was traced down to the fimbriated end to ensure that this was the fallopian tube. This was performed on the right side. The midportion of the fallopian tube was grasped again with Babcock clamp and it was ligated twice with two #2 plain absorbable sutures. The loop was cut away with Metzenbaum scissors and hemostasis was performed with the electrocautery. After completion of the operation on the right fallopian tube, the two severed ends of tube were placed back into the peritoneum so as to have a tendency to retract from one another.

The process was repeated on the opposite side, grasping the midportion of the left fallopian tube and following it to the fimbriated end to guarantee that this was the fallopian tube. The midportion was again grasped and the loop being held up was ligated with two #2 plain absorbable sutures. The loop was cut away with Metzenbaum scissors and the fallopian tube placed back into the peritoneum following excellent hemostasis. The peritoneum and fascia were reapproximated in the usual continuous fashion utilizing #2-0 _____ and the skin was reapproximated with subcuticular stitch using _____ . The patient's incision was cleaned and bandaid was placed over the incision. The patient tolerated the procedure well and was sent to the Recovery Room in good condition.

UCHIDA MINI-LAP STERILIZATION

Technique

After the patient was placed in the supine position, and also in modified lithotomy position, the patient was prepped and draped in the usual manner for vaginoabdominal procedure. Following placement of the uterine manipulator in the endometrial cavity, a 1 cm suprapubic incision was made and carried down to the fascia. The fascia and peritoneum were entered and the uterine fundus was maneuvered forward by the manipulator in the uterine cavity. A Babcock clamp was then used to deliver the fallopian tube through the small incision. The right fallopian tube was located first. At its midpoint, the mesosalpinx was dissected from the overlying muscular tube. This was accomplished by injecting a sufficient amount of saline-epinephrine solution at the tubo-mesosalpingeal junction to produce ballooning of the mesosalpinx. An avascular portion of the mesosalpinx was incised with Metzenbaum scissors. The muscular tube was then grasped through this incision with the clamp and delivered into a loop, and the tube was divided. Serosa from the proximal end was stripped back by blunt dissection. A 3–5 cm segment of the fallopian tube was excised leaving only a small stump. This proximal stump was ligated with a #2 nonabsorbable suture twice and allowed to fall back between the ballooned leaves of the broad ligament. The distal stump was then ligated and the edge of the broad ligament was closed with a suture of #3-0 _____ that terminated with a purse-string suture around the free end of the distal tube. The suture was tied so that the distal end of the fallopian tube projected into the abdominal cavity.

The same procedure that was performed on the right fallopian tube was performed on the left fallopian tube. The incision was closed in routine manner. Counts were correct and the patient tolerated the procedure well. Estimated blood loss was minimal. The patient went to the Recovery Room in good condition.

Suction dilatation and evacuation

Technique

Patient was prepped and draped in the usual manner for dilatation and evacuation. A weighted speculum was place into the vagina and a straight tenaculum was used on the anterior lip of the cervix. The dilators were placed into the cervical canal until a 3 mm dilatation had been reached. A small, curved, (#6, #7, #8, etc.) suction tip was then placed into the intrauterine cavity and the intrauterine cavity was suctioned thoroughly in systematic fashion. Contents were retrieved and a small malleable serrated curette was used following the suction curettage. This was performed until the intrauterine cavity was felt to be smooth and empty. Bleeding was minimal and the uterus firmed up nicely. A sponge stick with a single 4 x 4 sponge was placed into the vagina and held against the cervix following the removal of all instruments. After approximately 45 seconds this was removed and the area was inspected and found to be in excellent hemostatic condition. The patient tolerated the procedure well and all instrumentation was removed and counts were correct. The patient was sent to Recovery Room in good condition.

Vulvectomy

Technique

After the patient has been properly prepped and draped, the groin dissection was started with two teams. The groin incision was extended in an arcuate fashion from each anterior iliac superior crest, passing 2 cm above the symphysis and inguinal ligament. The butterfly vulvar incision includes the skin over the region of the fossa ovalis. The incision was extended inferiorly along the lateral aspect of the labia majora so as to remove all of the perineal body and tissue around the superior aspect of the anus. The skin and subcutaneous fat, including Camper's and Scarpa's fascia, were dissected to remove the superficial lymphatic channels and to avoid necrosis of skin margins. The incision was modified along the _____ (labiocrural folds, clitoris, or where ever the tumor is near) so that the incision extended for at least 2 cm beyond the tumor margins.

The lateral incision was extended to the fascia lata. The superior incision was made so as to remove all the lymphatic and areolar tissue down to the oponeurosis of the external oblique and anterior rectus fascia. Dissection was continued from the lateral aspect of the inguinal ligament to the region of the mons pubis.

The femoral sheath was incised along the medial margin of the sartorius muscle and along the lateral side of the artery. The femoral artery was palpated for identification and the femoral nerve was identified adjacent to it. The cribriform fascia was completely dissected off the artery and the external pudendal artery was carefully identified and ligated. The proximal end of the saphenous vein was transfixed and doubly ligated with _____ suture. The femoral sheath was dissected medially as an en bloc procedure.

The distal segment of the saphenous vein was ligated and excised as the dissection was continued toward the inner thigh.

Vulvar dissection was continued to include the perineal skin along the lateral side of the anus, a major portion of each labia, and along the periosteum of the symphysis at the level of the fascia of the deep musculature of the urogenital diaphragm. Thus, the bulbocavernosus, ischiocavernosus, and superficial transverse perinei muscles were removed.

The internal pudendal vessels were ligated with _____ suture as these were identified emerging from Alcock's canal at the 4 and 8 o'clock positions.

The vaginal incision was carried out proximal to the external urethral meatus circumscribing the introitus just outside the carunculae hymenoles. The mucosa of the lateral and posterior vaginal walls were undermined with _____ scissors for approximately 3 to 4 cm to form a mucosal flap for anastomosis to the perianal and vulvar skin. The vulva was removed after difficult but careful ligation of the blood supply to the clitoris making certain there were no retracted vessels beneath the inferior pubic ligament. The periurethral fascia was anchored to the subcutaneous fat at the lateral skin margins and the urethra was sutured securely to the skin margins beneath the symphysis with _____ suture.

Vulvar incision was closed by slightly undermining the thigh skin flaps and outer vaginal mucosa. The thigh/vulva flaps were sutured to the vaginal mucosa with a series of vertical mattress stitches of #0 _____ (delayed absorbable) suture. Care was taken to avoid as much tension as possible during closure.

Estimated blood loss was _____ . Sponge, instrument, needle, and lap counts were correct. _____ drains were attached to closed-suction (if drains were left). The patient went to the recovery room in _____ condition.

Author's note

Transcribe inguinal node dissection if performed and include description of drain placements if necessary.

Remember that if tumor is near the urethra or along the medial aspect of the labia minora – the outer one-third of the urethra should be removed and described. If cystourethrocele is present, plication and retropubic elevation of the urethrovesical angle would be necessary to avoid urinary incontinence and should also be described.

Each vulvectomy must be individualized according to whether simple, radical, separate incisions, unilateral or even exenteration would need to be performed depending on depth of stromal invasion, tumor size, and location of tumor. 5500 rads of midpelvic megavoltage pelvic irradiation might be recommended versus further deep node dissection and transcription depending upon evidence of groin metastasis. The author presently refers this surgery to oncology services secondary to lack of facilities and consultation in his rural area. This procedure is included for the benefit of residents and interns.